MIGRAINE

D0769991

MIGRAINE

Identify Your Triggers, Break Dependence on Medication, Take Back Your Life

AN INTEGRATIVE SELF-CARE PLAN FOR WELLNESS

Sharron Murray, MS, RN

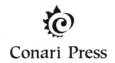

Conari Press

First published in 2013 by Conari Press, an imprint of
Red Wheel/Weiser, LLC
With offices at:
665 Third Street, Suite 400
San Francisco, CA 94107
www.redwheelweiser.com

Library of Congress Cataloging-in-Publication Data
    Murray, Sharron E.
    Migraine : identify your triggers, break your dependence on medica-
tion, take back your life : an integrative self-care plan for wellness / Sharron
E. Murray, MS, RN.
        pages cm
    Includes bibliographical references and index.
    ISBN 978-1-57324-595-1
    1. Migraine--Popular works. 2. Migraine--Alternative treatment--Pop-
ular works. 3. Self-care, Health--Popular works. I. Title.

    RC392.M92 2013
    616.8'4912--dc23

                                    2013000159

Interior by Frame25 Productions

Printed in the United States of America

WOR
10 9   8 7 6 5 4 3 2 1

The paper used in this publication meets the minimum requirements of
the American National Standard for Information Sciences—Permanence of
Paper for Printed Library Materials Z39.48-1992 (R1997).

To my husband, David

For loving me through sickness and in health and supporting me in everything I do. You are the half that makes me whole.

The greatest wealth is health.
　　—Virgil

Contents

Foreword

Pain is a dreaded human experience. It is said that most people make choices in life to either seek pleasure or avoid pain. For people with chronic debilitating pain, the pain robs them of the pleasures and quality of life. This is especially true with people who suffer from migraine.

In nearly 30 years of caring for patients with acupuncture and Chinese medicine, I've seen firsthand how during an acute attack the lives of my migraine patients simply stop. Alone in a dark room, they suffer with indescribable pain, dizziness, vision loss, nausea, and vomiting, praying for an end to the episode, and sometimes, in moments of despair, an end to it all.

Thank goodness for medication and thank goodness for acupuncture, for these have been the salvation for many of my migraine patients. Sharron Murray is one such patient who relentlessly sought out cures from East and West and found relief at last with integration of both.

Her journey was one of open-minded exploration. Expanding beyond her comfort zone and the boundaries of conventional Western medicine into Eastern medicine, and moving from a focus on disease to a focus on her whole self and ultimately her life, she found ways to address the physical as well as the mental and spiritual all at once.

Along the way, Sharron discovered that healing comes from within and that patients must take responsibility for their own health and that doctors are guides to activate the inner healer in each one of us.

With a background as a registered nurse and former college professor, which abundantly equipped her to teach and share complex medical subjects in an easy-to-digest format, Sharron has shared her triumphant story in a successful self-help regimen that she has put together as a self-care plan geared to assist other sufferers achieve wellness. The book is a meticulously researched, easy to understand, and essential resource that I am certain will help millions of migraine sufferers take back their lives.

—Dr. Mao Shing Ni
Author of *Secrets of Longevity* and *Secrets of Self-Healing*
and cofounder of Tao of Wellness and Yo San University of
Traditional Chinese Medicine (*www.taoofwellness.com*)

Acknowledgments

There are two people I must thank for helping me gain control of my life and my disease. First, Dr. Richard Byrd, my internist, who started me on a path to wellness by making me confront my dependence on medication. Second, Dr. Mao Shing Ni, who taught me that healing comes from within and one must take responsibility for his/her own health.

I have been blessed to have the support of both doctors as they worked with me over the years to help me achieve the mental, physical, and spiritual wellness I now enjoy.

As well, I thank both doctors for taking time from their busy schedules to review the manuscript as I wrote each chapter, and for sharing their knowledge and offering encouragement. A special thank-you to Dr. Mao Shing Ni for guiding me through my journey into Eastern medicine and for contributing the Foreword to this book.

I extend a special thank-you to Caroline Pincus. Her expertise as an editor has brought this book to life and enabled me to share the contents with you, my fellow migraineurs, as a self-care plan. It is my greatest wish that, as you read through the pages, you gain the inspiration and knowledge you need to plot your own path to wellness.

Introduction

Migraine, a genetic, neurological disease, affects the lives of millions of people worldwide. For many of us, the majority being women, the relentless headache, a symptom of the disease, is excruciating and accompanied by debilitating bouts of nausea and vomiting.

Without a cure, or "magic pill," thank goodness researchers and experts continue to focus on the physiological cause of our disease and the best medications to treat our headaches and nausea. However, medication, as I've found out, is not the only answer.

The disease involves much more than our heads and stomachs. It affects our bodies, minds, and spirits. In the throes of a severe attack, often during the very busiest years of our lives (twenties to fifties) when we're balancing our jobs, family responsibilities, and social obligations, our existence stops. Swallowing whatever drugs we can keep down, we're confined to a dark room until the episode is over. Feelings of helplessness and loss of control are prevalent.

Like me, you may have become a victim of medication overuse and rebound headaches because the drugs you take, whether over-the-counter (OTC) or prescription, allow you to make it through these horrific episodes and function as a spouse, partner, parent, aunt or uncle, cook, housekeeper, employee, stay-at-home parent, or friend. Unfortunately, just like me, to maintain the roles you juggle and keep on with the demands of your life, you may have been reluctant, or unable, to acknowledge your dependence on medication, change your lifestyle, take time for yourself, and reduce the effects the stress you impose on yourself has on your body.

After suffering from migraine headaches since I was five years old, and running on fumes for too many years to count, I managed to make it until my early fifties before I was forced to take responsibility for my life and my disease. In the years prior, I had been diagnosed with hypothyroidism in my twenties and, in my forties, a severe neck injury, along with mitral valve prolapse, a condition in which the valve between the upper and lower chambers on the left side of the heart does not close properly. In addition, I suffered from severe bouts of endometriosis and frequent episodes of sinusitis. All of these disorders magnified my migraine attacks, and the headaches were so horrific that many times I prayed to God that if he was going to take me, make it quick.

Thank goodness, in my early forties, I was referred to a migraine clinic. I learned about triggers (things that set off a migraine), how to deep breathe and meditate, and was told to pace myself. The designer drug, Imitrex, had just been introduced, and I took part in a clinical trial. To my delight, I discovered that if I took Imitrex each time I sensed a migraine on the horizon, I could get up at 4 a.m., make it to the hospital and teach students two days a week; and on the remaining days, plan and deliver lectures be it for a class or a consultant opportunity, travel across the city to gather research for a tenured professor, complete my graduate studies, finish my thesis, fulfill my obligations as a wife, and host a number of guests, including my nieces who often stayed for long periods of time and my nephews and their friends, all without drowsiness or nausea. For a few years, I thought I had my miracle cure.

So much for pacing myself. I joined the faculty at my university full time, added another load to my wagon, and embarked on a new opportunity. I signed a contract to write a book with a colleague about critical care nursing. She was in the middle of her doctoral degree and had a full teaching load. Well, I thought, if she can, why not me?

I crashed. I couldn't do it. I took more and more Imitrex to combat the headaches and still was unable to keep up the pace. As much as I loved teaching and my students, I left faculty to complete the book. By the time the book was published, instead of taking two or three Imitrex pills a month, I was up to eighteen Imitrex pills a month, plus injections and an inhaler when because of the dampness on the coast where I lived and the effect we thought the moisture had on my sinuses, my husband and I moved to the desert.

At the age of fifty-four, my move to the desert was the beginning of the events that would change my life. First, I met Dr. Richard Byrd (whom I refer to as Dr. B.), an internist who to this day remains my primary physician. After hearing the amount of medication I was taking, he shook his head and told me I had to reduce my dependence on Imitrex. With my background in critical care nursing, I knew he was right. However, the thought of giving up the only drug that had allowed me to function as a normal human being put me into a state of panic.

A few weeks later, I had the worst rebound migraine ever. Close to a seizure, I terrified my husband. Trembling, vomiting, and near collapse, I was half-carried by my husband into Dr. B.'s office for help.

As horrible as the episode was, the event turned out to be one of the best things that has ever happened to me. For months, my husband had begged me to try acupuncture, but I was skeptical. Then one morning, I met a neighbor who told me about a doctor who had saved her life in her late twenties, when she had a terrible respiratory illness. She urged me to go and see him about my migraines.

That is how I met Dr. Mao Shing Ni (whom I refer to as Dr. Mao). From Dr. B., I learned that medication is not the only answer. From Dr. Mao I learned that the key to wellness lies in the ability to accept responsibility for one's own health.

In taking back my life, I took two major steps. I'd always thought a migraine was a "really bad headache" I had to put up with because I couldn't cope with stress. Sound familiar? When I found out it was a disease, as I mentioned in the beginning of the Introduction, and the headache was only a symptom of the disease, the first step was to educate myself.

Given my nature and my academic background, I waded through the most recent evidence and research proposed by experts and professionals in the medical field about the illness. As well, because I had started acupuncture treatments and was curious to know how they worked, I studied the philosophy of Traditional Chinese Medicine (TCM) and the views about migraine disease held by doctors who practice TCM. I also became a student of healing touch, an energy-based healing practice that evolved from Eastern medicine and, like acupuncture, promotes self-healing through harmony and balance in the body's energy system, which I talk about in more detail in Chapter Nine.

The second step was to incorporate the guidelines and suggestions I had gathered through my research and from these experts and professionals into a personal wellness plan. As long as I've stuck to my wellness plan, for the past six years, I've been ninety-eight percent free of any headache, including the dreaded migraine.

In this book, I show you how, using these guidelines and suggestions, you can develop your own wellness plan and reduce the frequency and severity of your migraine attacks, break the cycle of medication dependence, consume a minimal amount of medication, and have control over your migraines, treatment, and your life. At this point, you may want to ask me, as many people have, "Why can't I just use your plan?"

Another thing I have found out: Migraineurs (those of us who suffer from migraine disease) are unique in our symptoms and the triggers that precipitate our attacks. For example, you may have a friend who gets a migraine attack only once a year and has some nausea, but nothing severe. You, on the other hand, may get migraine attacks two, three, four, or more times a month and be violently ill. Your friend may be fine with an OTC medication. You, however, may have to see a doctor for one or more prescription medications. As well, while a majority of us are affected by altitude and weather changes, food and beverage triggers like chocolate, cheese, alcohol, and caffeine may bother me, but not you. So, although I will share my wellness plan with you, trust me, as you read through the book, you will come across a number of other reasons that will not only make you want to, but also be excited to, develop your own personalized plan.

To help you out, I divided the book into four parts. The first part is devoted to Western medicine and the conventional approach to diagnosis and treatment of migraine disease. Once you understand the cause of the disease, where it comes from, why you have it, and what precipitates the attacks, you'll find that you're better prepared to manage your disease.

To achieve that goal, I explain theories proposed by the medical community about migraine disease, including what happens to the brain, blood vessels, and surrounding tissues during a migraine attack. This includes a discussion about the sympathetic nervous system and how stress, although not considered a trigger by many sources, plays a significant role in migraine attacks. Next I discuss primary and secondary headache types and the impact of injuries and diseases that may occur alongside migraine disease. Then I address common triggers and share with you how they cause our bodies to respond the crazy way they do, and relate how analgesic, abortive, and preventive (prophylactic) drug therapies can be used safely and effectively to manage our symptoms and in some cases prevent attacks.

In the second part, I explain the philosophy of Traditional Chinese Medicine (TCM) in health and natural healing and the views about migraine disease held by doctors who practice TCM. Whether or not you decide to see a doctor of TCM, a knowledge of Eastern medicine will help you understand how techniques like acupuncture, meditation, and mind-body exercises like tai chi can be incorporated into your healthcare plan to help reduce the effects of stress and avert headaches.

In the third part, I explore integrative therapies common to conventional Western medicine, TCM, and Holistic (body, mind, and spirit) Nursing and Medicine. Keeping in mind that what works for one person may not work for another, I include a discussion on the benefits of a number of therapies. These include physical therapy, chiropractic therapy, and exercise, as well as other techniques that have proven to be effective in the treatment of migraine disease such as yoga, meditation, breathing techniques, biofeedback, cold therapy, massage, reflexology, Reiki, and healing touch.

The fourth part reviews what you've learned in each chapter. If ways to begin your path to wellness have not already come to you, a recap will help you plot your course. In addition, I provide you with a number of resources to keep your knowledge of migraine disease updated and, should you require, to find a headache doctor and a licensed, or certified, practitioner in your area of treatments such as acupuncture, massage, and energy-healing techniques like healing touch and Reiki.

Lastly, the therapies I discuss in this book are not meant to take the place of conventional Western medicine. They are options you can explore, and combine, to enhance your personal pursuit of wellness. I believe the best healthcare plan is an integrative approach to wellness (not alternative approaches to health care where you choose one form of treatment over another). I think of an integrative approach as a collaborative program. Doctors of Western medicine or TCM, as well as Wellness practitioners, are guides to assist you in your path to wellness. The responsibility for healing lies within you and a personal commitment to your goals.

Happy Healing!

PART ONE

||||||||||||||||||||||||||||||||||||||||||||||||||||||||||||||||||||||||||||||||||||||||||||||||||||||||||||||||

Conventional Western Medicine and Migraine Disease

||||||||||||||||||||||||||||||||||||||||||||||||||||||||||||||||||||||||||||||||||||||||||||||||||||||||||||||||

CHAPTER ONE

Understanding Migraine Disease

In the last few decades, research about migraine headaches has come a long way. For example, a migraine headache is now believed to be a symptom of a more complex disorder, migraine disease. A number of theories have been proposed to explain the cause of our disease. Let's take a look at some of them.

The Vascular Theory

For much of my life, medical researchers believed migraine was a headache related to changes in the blood vessels in and around our brains. When exposed to triggers, which I explained in the Introduction as events capable of provoking our migraine attacks, our arteries narrowed. This constriction reduced blood flow and oxygen delivery to our tissues. As our constricted arteries expanded and tried to gain more oxygen, fluid leaked into the surrounding tissue and chemicals such as prostaglandin, which enhances the sensitivity of pain endings and stimulates the release of inflammatory agents, were released. This was known as the vascular theory.

Recent Theories

Recent theories suggest that migraine is a neurological disease, which involves more than dilation and constriction of blood vessels. Evidence suggests we have an inherited disruption in brain function that makes our brain cells more excitable than others. When exposed to triggers capable of provoking a migraine attack, a chemical imbalance occurs in our brains. Levels of neurotransmitters (chemical messengers that pass information from one cell to another), such as glutamate, serotonin, dopamine, and norepinephrine, are altered. The most recent theories implicate one or more of these neurotransmitters as culprits in our disease. So, what are these recent theories?

Cortical Spreading Depression Theory

The cortical spreading depression theory believes that a wave of hyperexcitability spreads across the outer layer of our brain (the cortex), followed by a period of suppression. When brain activity is depressed, inflammatory mediators are released. These inflammatory mediators irritate the cranial nerve roots, in particular the trigeminal nerve, which conveys sensory information for much of our head and face.

Glutamate, a neurotransmitter present in the trigeminal nerve, is thought to play a role in the cortical spreading depression. As well, a neurotransmitter found in the brain and spinal cord and known as substance P is thought to coexist with glutamate. Substance P is believed to be involved with the inflammatory process, vasodilation, smooth muscle contraction, nausea and vomiting, regulation of mood disorders such as anxiety, and the sensation of pain.

The Serotonin Theory

Serotonin, also known as hydroxytryptamine or 5-HT, is believed to have a major role in migraine disease. The serotonin theory suggests that we have a defect in a specific type of serotonin receptor that causes our blood vessels to constrict, or narrow. As a result, in the presence of certain triggers, arteries that supply blood to our brain dilate, or expand. The dilation, or stretching, of the arteries in and around our brain causes fluid to leak into surrounding tissue. The fluid leak damages tissue cells and stimulates the release of inflammatory agents, which contribute to the swelling of the arteries and surrounding tissue, leads to irritation of nerves, and intensifies our throbbing pain. Also, because serotonin enhances endorphins (a natural analgesic found in the gray matter of the brain) and has an effect on substance P, low levels of serotonin further exacerbate our pain.

Besides alterations in cerebral blood flow and the sensation of pain, changes in the levels of serotonin are thought to be responsible for a number of gastrointestinal symptoms such as nausea, vomiting, and diarrhea that many of us experience during an attack. This is because serotonin is also a neurotransmitter for the enteric nervous system, or ENS, which is located in the abdomen (ninety-five percent of the body's serotonin is located in the gut). Often referred to as the *second brain* or *gut brain,* the ENS causes contraction of the smooth muscle of the gut that is important for normal digestion and the movement of food through the intestines (peristalsis). As well, it regulates intestinal blood flow, the transport of mucosal water and electrolytes, and propulsive bowel function.

Blood levels of dopamine and norepinephrine are believed to fluctuate with our serotonin levels. All three of these neurotransmitters may be responsible for many of the other symptoms we exhibit as our migraine attack progresses. For instance, high levels of serotonin may make us feel calm, full, relaxed, and even drowsy. Low levels may cause us to feel anxious, irritable, and depressed. They may also promote food cravings for starches and sugars, like crackers, chips, ice cream, and chocolate.

An increase in dopamine and norepinephrine levels may make us feel more energetic, focused, and alert. A decrease in these levels may contribute to the fatigue, inability to concentrate, yawning, nausea, and vomiting many of us experience.

The Integrated, or Unifying, Theory

The integrated or unifying theory suggests that both vascular and neural influences cause the pain associated with migraine headaches. This theory suggests that stress and other triggers cause changes in the levels of epinephrine in our bodies, which affects serotonin levels. Fluctuations in serotonin levels cause blood vessels to constrict and dilate. Chemicals, such as substance P, are released and further irritate nerves and blood vessels and enhance our pain and inflammation.

Defining Migraine Disease

The organization MAGNUM (Migraine Awareness Group: A National Understanding for Migraineurs) refers to migraine as an organic neurological disease. Although the importance of the role of one theory over another is debatable in the literature, the disease itself seems to be related to a complex series of events that results in a breakdown of communication between the neurotransmitters in our brain and, as more recent research suggests, in our gut. When exposed to controllable or uncontrollable triggers, which you read about in Chapter Three, a chain reaction is initiated that sets off a cascade of events referred to as a *migraine attack*.

What Is a Migraine Attack?

A migraine attack is the episodic event we endure in the presence of an appropriate trigger. The attack has been split into four phases: the *prodrome, aura, headache,* and *postdrome.* Not all of us go through each phase. For instance, you may never have a prodrome or an aura. Other migraineurs may have a migraine attack without a headache. A migraine attack may last for several hours. Let's take a look at these phases.

Prodrome Phase

Anywhere from forty to sixty percent of us have warning signs that may present a few hours or up to two days prior to the onset of a headache. Our symptoms reflect fluctuations in the blood levels of the neurotransmitters and endorphins I just discussed.

In my case, a couple of days before the headache would break, I would have a period of hyperactivity and feel on top of the world. Then I would become irritable and so fatigued that it was difficult to hold my head up. I would have an increased sensitivity to light and sound, which made it difficult for me to watch TV or go to a movie. My neck became stiff and painful, and I craved salty foods like soda crackers. My face, eyelids, and abdomen would swell and remained swollen until the migraine subsided. My husband would take one look at me and say, "You are going to have a migraine." He became so familiar with the sight, he was able to tell his secretary, who also suffered from migraines, she was going to have an attack and send her home.

You may relate to some of these symptoms or have others including

- Agitation

- Change of appetite (anorexia)

- Difficulty in concentration

- Drowsiness

- Depression (become withdrawn)

- Diarrhea or constipation

- Euphoria (feeling high)

- Food cravings (sweet, fat, and salty)

- Slurred or rapid speech

- Thirst

- Yawning

Aura Phase

Approximately twenty percent of us have an aura that develops over five to sixty minutes prior to a headache. The symptoms, thought to be related to the cortical spreading depression theory I previously discussed, may occur in isolation or precede or accompany the headache phase. They should disappear with the end of our aura, or migraine, and may include

- **Changes in the way we see:** For instance, flashing, zigzagged, or brightly colored lights that progress outward from the center of our visual field. Or a blind spot or hole in our visual field. On occasion, I've experienced a hole in my visual field accompanied by brightly colored, zigzagged lights and found the experience to be most alarming. More often, for me, blurred vision was a sure sign a migraine was on my horizon.

- **Changes in sensation:** For example, pins and needles on the hand and arm on one side of our body, or around our nose and mouth on the same side of the body. Or we may have prickly or burning sensations, or muscle weakness, on one side of our body. *A word of caution:* It's important to note that motor deficits and paralysis are rare and an indication for you to seek immediate medical attention.

- **Changes in hearing:** For instance, we may hear music playing or a clock ticking.

- **Changes in smell or taste:** For me, another sure sign of an impending migraine is the smell of cigarette smoke, even though no one around me has a lighted cigarette.

- **Changes in the way we speak:** For example, we may speak incorrectly, or be unable to recall the words we want to say. In my case, I would speak so fast that I would trip over the words I wanted to say. Many times, in particular when I was giving a lecture, my audience was forced to ask me to slow down.

Headache Phase

The intense, throbbing pain typically associated with migraine headaches may be on one side of our head (unilateral), both sides of our head (bilateral), or behind our eyes. Our pain may be aggravated by light, noise, and odors. An increase in physical activity may exacerbate the pain or, in some cases, may relieve our agony. The accompanying symptoms, again, may be related to fluctuations in the blood levels of neurotransmitters and endorphins. The headache may last from four to seventy-two hours, or sometimes longer.

In my case, the associated symptoms like nausea and vomiting were as debilitating as my headache. I was trapped. Tied to my bed afraid to move, not a single digit, finger or toe, lest I had to dash to the bathroom and hang over the toilet bowl until the retching that threatened to blow my head apart stopped. In between the bouts of vomiting, I'd lie beneath a heavy load of blankets and shiver with cold. To make it worse, I had a continuous nasal drip and nasal congestion so severe that I had to breathe with my mouth hanging open, and if I should be lucky enough to fall asleep, wake up with my tongue glued to the top of my mouth and gasping for water.

Again, sound familiar? You may relate to the nausea and vomiting, shivering, runny nose (rhinorrhea), and dehydration, or have other symptoms, which may include

- Confusion

- Diarrhea

- Fluid retention

- Food cravings

- Hot flashes

- Inability to concentrate

- Irrational emotions such as fear, depression, nervousness, anxiety, and panic

- Loss of appetite

- Sensitivity to touch (allodynia), sound (phonophobia), and light (photophobia)

- Tearing of one or both eyes (lacrimation)

Postdrome Phase

After all that, the migraine is not over. For some of us, it may take hours, others days, before a hangover effect disappears. The symptoms we experience are often attributed to the medications we've ingested to stop the pain and vomiting but, again, may be related to those pesky neurotransmitters and inflammatory agents. As I did, you may feel drained of energy, have a low-grade headache and sometimes a reoccurrence of the headache.

Fatigue, irritability, and tender and sore muscles of the head, face, and neck may also be bothersome.

A Word About the Nervous System

The nervous system is composed of the central nervous system (CNS) and the peripheral nervous system (PNS). The CNS is made up of the nerves in the brain and spinal cord. The PNS is divided into the autonomic and voluntary nervous systems. The voluntary nervous system allows us to control movement of the muscular and skeletal systems. The autonomic nervous system is divided into the sympathetic and parasympathetic systems.

The sympathetic system is our "fight or flight" primitive response to pain, danger, or stress. The parasympathetic system is our slow down, or relaxation, response that lowers heart rate and blood pressure and regulates digestion. The enteric nervous system (ENS), which I discussed earlier, is believed to be associated with, although somewhat independent from, the parasympathetic nervous system.

It's important for you to understand that often our migraine attacks can activate our sympathetic nervous system. Besides increasing levels of norepinephrine in the blood, levels of epinephrine (a hormone secreted from the adrenal glands) are increased. I talk more about these hormones and the stress response in Chapter Three, but for now you need to know that this increase in norepinephrine and epinephrine constricts blood vessels; shunts blood from the skin, kidney, and digestive organs to the heart, brain, and skeletal muscles; and raises our heart rate, blood pressure, and blood sugar.

Because gastric emptying is delayed, the oral medications we take are prevented from entering the small intestine and being absorbed. Hence no matter how many pills we swallow, they may not work. Accompanying symptoms to this sympathetic response may include facial pallor, cold hands and feet, chills, nausea and vomiting, diarrhea, restlessness, insomnia, palpitations, dry mouth, headache, light headedness, rapid speech, stuttering, nervousness, irritability, confusion, forgetfulness, anxiety, and panic attacks.

Looking Back and Glimpsing Ahead

In this chapter, you discovered a variety of theories offered by the medical community to explain the cause of migraine disease. You also learned about the role of the sympathetic nervous system in our disorder.

Now that you understand what is happening to your body during a migraine attack, you can apply the knowledge you have gained in the chapters ahead. For example:

- You will see how balancing your serotonin levels by avoiding your food and beverage triggers and incorporating integrative therapies like acupuncture, meditation, and exercise into your wellness plan can minimize many of the symptoms you experience during your migraine attack.

- You will discover how to curb, or turn off, your sympathetic nervous system and decrease your body's physiologic response to stress, which I talk about in detail in Chapter Three, as well as other chapters throughout the book.

- You will have a better grasp of how the medications we look at in Chapter Four can help to relieve, abort, or prevent your headache.

CHAPTER TWO

Why You Have Migraine Disease

IN THE INTRODUCTION, I told you migraine was a genetic, neurological disease. In Chapter One, you looked at the medical
theories offered to explain the cause of our disease. Now, you
need to examine the genetic relationship.

Although research suggests migraine is a genetically based
disease, exact genetics have not been identified. Some sources
believe there may be a gene that causes a decrease in serotonin
production. Other reports indicate there may be an abnormality
in a gene that inhibits the function of a protein called TRESK.
TRESK is thought to control nerve cell excitability and the sensation of pain in an area of nerves at the base of the brain (see the
"References" section at the end of the book for further information).

While research continues to attempt to link specific genes
to the cause of migraines, one thing is known: If one of your
parents suffers, or suffered, from migraine disease, there is a fifty
percent chance you may as well. Also, the inherited tendency
may be passed from another family member, such as a grandpar-
ent, aunt, or uncle.

Looking back at my family history, I don't recall either of my parents suffering from migraine disease. However, I have many memories of my father sitting at the dining room table, with his head covered by a towel and his body bent over a bowl of steaming water, trying to relieve the horrible sinus headaches he experienced, which, when I think about it, could have been misdiagnosed. Currently, although I do not have my own children, I have two nieces and a great-nephew who have migraine disease and, like me, started to have the headaches at a young age.

Frequency of Migraine Disease

While almost everyone gets a headache sometime in their lives, you may not realize that migraine disease is the second most common cause of headaches. The disease occurs worldwide and affects more than thirty million people in the United States. Of these, approximately two-thirds are females and one-third are males. White women have the highest incidence of migraine disease in the United States. Attacks often begin in childhood (most of us experience attacks before twenty years of age) and increase in prevalence up to forty or fifty years of age, and then may decline. Boys are affected slightly more than girls in the early years, and then with the onset of menarche (first period), female predominance occurs.

Diagnosing Migraine Disease

I'm surprised at how many people tell me about their headaches but have not seen a doctor for a diagnosis, or have been misdiagnosed. If you haven't seen a doctor for a diagnosis, now is the time to do so.

If you feel you may have been misdiagnosed, you may want to see a headache specialist. I finally did in my forties, when I went to a migraine clinic. If you don't have a migraine clinic in your area or cannot find a headache doctor, check out Chapter Ten where I provide a number of resources to assist you in your search.

In my case, I saw a variety of doctors and had various diagnoses before I made it to the migraine clinic. My first headache diagnosis took place the summer I was five years old. The weather was hot and dry, and while my sisters played outside, I was inside with a cold cloth over my eyes. Apparently this happened so often that my parents took me to our family doctor to address the issue. He ordered an electroencephalogram (EEG). I presume the EEG was normal as my parents were told I had sun stroke and to give me an aspirin and keep me out of the sun.

The diagnosis stuck all through my teens, and regardless of the weather, whenever I had a headache, my parents would say "sunstroke," and to bed I went with the aspirin. In my twenties, my diagnosis was changed to a tension headache, and for many years, I was given all sorts of medications, including sedatives, muscle relaxants, and combination pain relievers like Fiorinal. None of these drugs aborted my headaches. They only worsened my nausea and vomiting and made me drowsy.

Now that I have convinced you to make a medical appointment and shared with you the reasons why you may want to choose a physician who is familiar with headache medicine, let's look at what to expect in your first visit. At this time, your doctor should take a thorough history and perform a physical examination. The focus of the history will be on questions about your headache. Below, I have included some sample questions. You may want to write your answers down so you don't forget anything during your appointment.

How Old Were You When Your Headaches Began?

As I mentioned earlier in the chapter, migraine disease usually begins in childhood, adolescence, or the early twenties. For many women, the attacks increase after puberty and decline with the onset of menopause. In men, headaches often peak in their thirties and then decline. If your headaches have started later in your life, in addition to the physical exam, be prepared for your doctor to perform a thorough neurological exam to rule out other causes for your headaches.

How Often Do Your Headaches Occur?

Although some people may go many months without a headache, a migraine may occur from one to eight times per month, or more frequently if you have chronic migraine (see the upcoming "International Headache Society Classification of Headaches" section) or rebound headaches, which I talk about later in this chapter. It's important to tell your doctor if you have daily headaches as this will help your doctor distinguish between migraine disease, tension-type headaches (see "International Headache Classification of Headaches"), or a pattern of medication (prescription, or OTC) overuse.

Up to sixty percent of women who suffer from migraine disease say their migraine attacks are related to their menstrual cycle. I explain the relationship between hormones and migraine attacks in Chapter Three.

Where Is Your Pain Located?

A migraine headache may occur on one side of your head, both sides of your head, or change during your attack. The pain may also occur at your temples or back of your head. If you have a tension-type headache, along with your migraine, you may experience muscle tightening, or contraction, in the forehead, neck, shoulders, or skull.

How Long Do Your Headaches Last?

A migraine attack usually lasts from four to seventy-two hours. If you have an attack that lasts longer than seventy-two hours and is accompanied by severe nausea and vomiting, you may have what is known as *status migrainous* and require hospitalization to treat dehydration (see "International Headache Society Classification of Headaches").

How Do You Describe Your Pain?

The typical headache associated with a migraine attack is pulsating, throbbing, severe, and often incapacitating. Physical exertion may increase the severity. Other types of headache pain may be related to rare types of migraine, tension-type headaches, cluster headaches, and secondary headaches (see "International Headache Society Classification of Headaches").

Does Your Headache Interfere with Your Lifestyle?

The impact your headache has on your work, home, and family life helps your doctor determine whether you need aggressive therapy, such as prescription medications, or less aggressive, such as the OTC medications you most likely have already relied on to relieve your pain.

What Makes Your Pain Go Away?

A cold compress, a dark room, and sleep (especially in children) may help some people who experience the headache associated with migraine disease find relief (a cold gel pack is still my best friend). However, for the majority of people, either OTC or prescription medications are required to treat the symptoms.

I talk more about medications in Chapter Four and how important it is for your doctor to match the right kind of medication to your headache, but for now, take a look at why you don't want to take more drugs than you have to. As I mentioned in the Introduction, this is where I got into trouble. Because Imitrex stopped my headache and I could function, I took more than I should have. My body got used to the drug being there, and when I didn't take it, I got another headache. So, I took some more. Thus began my downward cycle of rebound headaches.

In other words, the Imitrex constricted my blood vessels so the pain stopped. But, when it wore off, my vessels expanded, and I got another headache, so I took another dose. Medications taken more than three times a week on a regular basis that may result in rebound headaches include acetaminophen, aspirin, ibuprofen, narcotics, barbiturates, sedatives, other migraine medications besides Imitrex, and those that contain caffeine.

What Other Symptoms Do You Have with Your Headache?

You may want to refer back to Chapter One where I discuss a number of symptoms that may occur with your migraine attack. The most common ones include nausea, vomiting, and sensitivity to light and/or sound.

Do You Have Any Warning Symptoms of an Impending Attack?

Again, you may want to refer back to Chapter One. Some people have an aura and/or prodrome; others do not.

Are You Able to Associate Your Migraine Attacks with Specific Triggers?

Your migraine attack may be initiated by one or more of the triggers I discuss in Chapter Three. Knowing and eliminating the things that set off your migraine attack can help reduce the frequency and severity of your attacks and reduce the amount of medication your doctor might prescribe.

Has There Been a Change in the Pattern of Your Headache in the Last Few Months?

Your doctor will want to establish a baseline for your headache pattern and associated symptoms. A change in the pattern helps your doctor order tests to rule out secondary headaches and comorbid diseases, which I discuss at the end of this chapter.

Following are some red flags that alert doctors to pursue further investigation, such as a urinalysis, extensive laboratory tests like blood chemistry and a liver profile (many medications are contraindicated if you have any signs of liver disease), an EEG (electroencephalogram), a CT scan, an MRI (magnetic resonance imaging), a lumbar puncture, or a spinal tap, where a needle is inserted and fluid is withdrawn from the lower area of your spine:

- Your worst headache ever.

- Pain that reaches peak intensity within seconds to minutes (known as a *thundercap headache* that feels like a blow to your head).

- A new onset of a headache after you reach fifty years of age.

- Abrupt onset of a headache with exertion, sexual activity, coughing, or sneezing.

- Your headache is accompanied by a fever, a stiff neck, or other signs of a bacterial or viral infection.

- You have focal neurological deficits such as papill-edema (a change in the optic disc of your eye suggestive of increased intracranial pressure), weakness in your arms or legs, memory loss, or sensory loss.

- *A word of caution:* If you have a new onset of numbness, loss of motor coordination, vision disturbances, speech disturbances, confusion, or any

other change in your level of consciousness, you
need to seek immediate medical help as you may
have a complication of migraine disease known as a
migraine stroke (see "International Classification of
Headaches").

As you can see, the more information you provide your
doctor, the better prepared your doctor will be to rule out
any underlying organic causes for your headaches, determine
whether you're suffering from more than one type of headache,
and provide an effective treatment plan for you. I've included
the following examples from my personal experience to further
illustrate this point.

I recall in my final year of my undergraduate degree that
three of my friends and I were sitting around the lunch table
and complaining about our headaches. Final exams were on the
horizon, papers were due on numerous subjects, one of us was
the mother of two boys, one recently married, and three of us
worked part time at the university hospital. At that time, we
didn't know anything about migraine disease and triggers; we'd
had headaches for years and just assumed we were overloaded
with stress.

Then the one recently married began to have projectile vomiting with her headaches and had to leave work on many occasions. She also had difficulty with her contact lenses, and on our
urging, went to her eye doctor to complain. He immediately saw
papilledema, which I described earlier, and sent her to a neurologist. He diagnosed her with an aggressive brain tumor.

Another example involves one of my sisters, who never had
a migraine-type headache until her forties. At that time, she
started to have episodic periods of hypertension accompanied
by such severe headaches that she became a frequent visitor to

the emergency department. Turns out, she had multiple sclerosis and her headaches were related to an undiagnosed disease.

I have another sister who never experienced headaches until she was involved in a car accident and received a severe whiplash injury. The resultant headaches were excruciating and not only did she become a frequent visitor to the emergency room, but also for a short period of time she ended up dependent on narcotics and a number of other prescription medications.

Because so many people suffer from headaches and headaches have numerous causes, many of which can be life-threatening, the International Headache Society (*www.ihs-headache.org*) developed a classification system (see next section and References at the end of the book) to help doctors provide accurate diagnoses and offer effective treatments for their patients. Much of the information can be confusing for doctors, as well as those of us who are patients, but I've included it for your reference, and because I've referred to it numerous times in this chapter. Doctors are cautioned to use the content as guidelines.

According to the International Headache Society, headaches are classified as primary or secondary. A primary headache is one that you may have in the absence of any underlying systemic, organ or vessel disease, bacterial or viral infection, or injury. In other words, your headache occurs in your otherwise healthy body (your neurological exam is normal).

Secondary headaches are caused by an underlying disorder. In other words, your headache is a symptom of another problem you might have, not a primary problem like it is in your migraine disease.

International Headache Society Classification of Headaches

Primary headaches include the following:

1. Migraine: Second most common type of headache.

1a) Types of migraine:

Migraine with aura: Two known attacks.

- Reversible aura symptoms.

- Aura develops over more than four minutes and lasts for less than sixty minutes.

- Headache follows aura within sixty minutes.

Migraine without aura: Pain is usually unilateral (one side of head), pulsating in quality, of moderate to severe intensity, and aggravated by physical activity.

- Associated symptoms include nausea and vomiting and sensitivity to light and/or sound; must have five attacks that fill the preceding criteria and no secondary headache disorder; headaches last four to seventy-two hours.

Chronic migraine: Occurs fifteen or more days per month.

- Characteristics same as migraine without aura; may or may not be associated with medication overuse (rebound headache).

1b) Rare types of migraine:

Basilar artery migraine: Dangerous as may lead to stroke or transient ischemic attack (TIA).

- Associated symptoms include dizziness, loss of balance, poor muscle coordination, double vision, slurred speech, numbness, severe vomiting.

- Previously thought to occur only in adolescent and young women, but now believed to occur in both sexes and all ages.

- Migraine-specific medications such as triptans and ergotamines are contraindicated.

Ocular or retinal migraine: Visual disturbances occur in only one eye and include flashing lights, dark spots, partial or complete loss of vision (temporary blindness).

- Last less than one hour.
- Headache may begin during visual disturbances and last from four hours to three days and may be accompanied by sensitivity to light and/or sound and nausea.
- Must have had two attacks to be diagnosed and normal eye exam between attacks.

Ophthalmoplegic migraine: Pain is centered around the eye and may be accompanied by droopy eyelid, double vision, and enlarged pupil.

Abdominal migraine: More common among younger children (older children may present with pain on one side of the skull, and the location and intensity may change between attacks).

- The midline abdominal pain or cramping may last from one to seventy-two hours.
- Associated symptoms may include nausea and vomiting and loss of appetite, paleness with dark circles beneath the eyes, sensitivity to light, sound, and smells, tearing, thirst, swollen nasal passages, and a need to sleep.
- Child usually has a family history of migraine and often develops traditional migraine as an adult.

Hemiplegic migraine: Usually genetic in nature but may occur in absence of family history.

- May develop during childhood.
- Symptoms begin ten to ninety minutes before the onset of headache.
- Along with temporary paralysis on one side of the body, may include vertigo (sensation of spinning), confusion, lack of limb coordination, nausea and vomiting, and vision disturbances.
- May have sudden onset and resemble stroke in appearance.

1c) Complications of migraine:

Migraine stroke (migrainous infarction): A stroke may be related to decreased blood flow to the brain (ischemic), or rupture of a blood vessel (hemmorrhagic).

- Risk is rare; however, factors such as smoking, oral contraceptives, hormone replacement therapy, high blood pressure, and elevated cholesterol make those with migraine disease more vulnerable *to* ischemic stroke.

- More common in migraine with aura and in those who have migraines over the age of sixty.

Status migrainous: Migraine lasting > 72 hours.

- Associated with severe nausea and vomiting, which may lead to dehydration and/or stroke.

- Hospitalization may be required to treat pain and replace fluid loss.

2. Tension-type headache: Most common type of headache.

- Associated with muscle tightening or contraction in the forehead, neck, shoulders, or skull.

- May occur in the presence of factors such as stress, poor posture, eye strain, lack of sleep; may coexist with migraine.

- Symptoms may include mild to moderate pain which is usually bilateral but may occur anywhere in the head.

- Pain described as a tightening or pressing rather than the throbbing quality of migraine.

- May be accompanied by sensitivity to light or sound, but not both; pain does not worsen with exertion; not accompanied by nausea or vomiting.

- Must have had ten previous headaches and no evidence of a secondary headache.

Chronic tension-type headache: Occurs on fifteen or more days per month.

- Characteristics similar to tension-type headaches; may, or may not, be associated with medication overuse.

3. **Cluster headache:** Least common type of headache.

- Excruciating pain which often centers around the eye and is unilateral (on one side).
- Related to stimulation of the main facial nerve (trigeminal); may last from 15 to 180 minutes.
- May be accompanied by any of the following symptoms: runny nose (rhinorrhea); teary eyes (lacrimation); swollen eyelids; contraction of the pupil (miosis) and drooping eyelid (ptosis); facial sweating; restlessness and agitation.
- No evidence of a secondary headache disorder.

    Hemicrania Continua: A continuous, unilateral headache with characteristics similar to cluster headache.

    - Pain must have periods of severity and present for one month.

4. **Chronic daily headache (CDH):** Headache of any kind that occurs more than fifteen days per month.

- Not associated with any structural lesion.

5. **New daily persistent headache:** Unremitting from onset.

- Mild to moderate intensity; pressing or tightening in quality.
- May have sensitivity to light and/or noise; may be accompanied by mild nausea.

Secondary headaches include the following:

- Head or neck injuries, including brain contusion, concussion, and whiplash
- Problems with the blood vessels of the head and neck, including aneurysms, carotid artery disease, stroke, and inflammation of the arteries
- Nonvascular issues of the brain, including brain tumor, increased cerebrospinal fluid pressure, seizures (epilepsy), medication overuse (rebound headaches), alcohol and drug abuse, and withdrawal from both
- Infections, including sinusitis, meningitis, encephalitis, pneumonia, and AIDS

- Disruptions in the body's homeostatic environment caused by conditions including hypertension, hypothyroidism, renal failure, dehydration, allergies, and sleep disorders
- Problems with the eyes, ears, nose, or throat, including temporomandibular disorder (TMD)
- Psychiatric disorders including depression, anxiety, and bipolar disorder

Secondary headaches should improve, or resolve, with treatment of the causative disorder. For example, my friend who was diagnosed with a brain tumor, whom I mentioned earlier, did have relief of her headache when the tumor was removed and the pressure in her skull decreased. As well, my sister, with the neck injury, whom I also mentioned earlier, had tremendous improvement in her headaches with aggressive physical therapy and a medication regimen that did not include narcotics.

At this point, it's important for you to note that, even though you may have been diagnosed with migraine disease, you can develop a secondary headache related to another disorder. Again, if your headache changes in any way, you need to make an appointment and talk to your doctor about your new symptoms so you can receive the help you require.

For example, I mentioned in the Introduction that I had a severe neck injury in my forties. Although I'd had migraine attacks since I was five years old, these headaches were different. The pain began at the base of my skull, spread to the top of my head, and magnified until I thought my head would blow off (I called them the "boomer"). The vomiting was nonstop, and my normal migraine medication was ineffective (mostly because I could not keep it down). A visit to my doctor and a subsequent MRI revealed that I had injured a disc in my neck through a fall off our deck. I'd been to the emergency room at the time of the fall, but because I'd split my toe wide open and cracked my elbow, and at the time, had no distress related to my neck, the injury was missed. After an intensive period of stretching exercises and physical therapy, which I have kept up for many years, and regular sessions of acupuncture, the "boomer" episodes have disappeared.

I also mentioned in the Introduction that I suffered from pounding sinus headaches for many years and was frequently diagnosed with episodes of sinusitis. Nasal sprays and antihistamines did not provide relief, instead causing rebound headaches. At one point, after a CT scan, a doctor suggested I have surgery to widen my nasal passages. A possible risk, he warned me, was blindness. Thank goodness, about that time, I started the migraine clinic and was told by my neurologist that I did not have sinusitis. Many people, I learned, believe they have sinus headaches because the symptoms, including congestion, pain behind the eyes, and in the forehead, are similar to the pain experienced during a migraine attack.

Another point for you to note is that you can still, as I do, have migraine disease and on occasion develop a secondary headache related to sinusitis. The distinction between the sinus component of a migraine headache and sinusitis is that sinusitis is caused by inflammation and/or infection of the lining of the sinuses. The pain may occur early in the morning, be worse when you bend over, cause your upper teeth to ache, and may be accompanied by fever, nasal discharge, or congestion. Unlike a migraine, which may last one to two days, the headache may last ten to fourteen days or longer. Treatment consists of plenty of fluids, a humidifier if you live in a dry climate, nasal irrigation to prevent bacteria from becoming trapped, nasal decongestants and, if necessary, antibiotics.

What Is a Comorbid Disease?

A comorbid (coexisting) disease is one that occurs alongside another disease at the same time, in the same person, with greater frequency than seen in the general population. Migraineurs, it appears, are more likely than non-migraineurs to have comorbid disorders. Remember though, just like the triggers I talk about in Chapter Three, even grouped as migraineurs, we're unique. You may develop one of these disorders during your lifetime, several of them, or none of them.

Although reports in the literature vary (and there are some gray areas), there is enough evidence to suggest that some of the disorders we experience in higher frequency than in the general population may include depression, anxiety, panic disorders, bipolar disorder, mitral valve prolapse, Raynaud's disease, hypertension, stroke (also a complication of migraine disease known as *migrainous infarction*), hypothyroidism, epilepsy, multiple sclerosis, lupus erythematosus (migraine with aura), endometriosis, irritable bowel syndrome, celiac disease, chronic fatigue syndrome, and asthma.

Possible explanations for the association between our migraine attacks and these diseases include alterations in the levels of neurotransmitters like serotonin and glutamate (for example, depression and epilepsy), decreased blood flow to the tissues (for example, hypertension and stroke), or genetic or familial tendencies (for example, hypothyroidism, mitral valve prolapse, and multiple sclerosis). If you want more details on any of these diseases, please refer to the "References" section at the end of this book.

It is important for you to understand that if you have one or more of these comorbid conditions, they can have a big impact on the frequency and severity of your migraine attacks. For instance, I mentioned in the Introduction that I was diagnosed with hypothyroidism in my early twenties. However, that was after I endured months of daily headaches and chronic fatigue. Because I suffered from migraine headaches, my doctor did not suspect that my increase in headaches might be related to another disease. Upon the urging of my father, who had been diagnosed with myxedema (an extreme form of hypothyroidism) the year prior, I had my doctor check my thyroid hormones. Once my hypothyroidism was diagnosed and treated, my daily headaches disappeared, although the migraines continued. Today, because a strong connection has been found between new daily persistent headache, chronic migraine, and hypothyroidism, some sources recommend that doctors evaluate thyroid function on all migraine patients.

Another personal example I mentioned in the Introduction was that I had been diagnosed with endometriosis in my thirties. My migraine headaches were worse at the time and thought to be hormonal. However, removal of my uterus in my mid-thirties and my ovaries in my forties, because of extensive cystic disease related to endometriosis and thought to be cancer, made no difference in the frequency or severity of my migraine headaches. Recent studies have shown that although the incidence of endometriosis is higher in women with migraine disease than those without, and both are influenced by ovarian hormones, the reasons for the increased association remain unclear.

Again, in my case, I mentioned in the Introduction that I was diagnosed with mitral valve prolapse in my forties. Similar to people with migraine disease whose brain cells are believed to be extremely sensitive to stimuli, people with mitral valve prolapse are thought to be wired differently. Exposure to normal stressors, such as weather or altitude changes, can flood the body with norepinephrine and epinephrine and cause a number of symptoms, including migraine headaches.

Another thing you need to know is that comorbid disorders may be masked, or difficult to diagnose, because of the role migraine disease plays in your life. However, once your comorbid conditions have been diagnosed, the treatment your doctor prescribes may not only help your comorbid disease but also your migraine attacks.

For example, an antidepressant medication may be helpful for migraineurs who suffer from depression, and an anticonvulsant drug may benefit migraineurs who have epilepsy, or in my sister's situation, those who have seizures associated with multiple sclerosis. For me, the calcium channel blocker I take for the palpitations and rapid heart rate related to my mitral valve prolapse doubles as a preventive medicine for my migraine attacks.

Looking Back and Glimpsing Ahead

In this chapter, you learned about the genetic relationship to migraine disease and the importance of a diagnosis for your headaches. As well, you discovered the need to provide your doctor with as much information as possible to facilitate an accurate diagnosis.

You also found out that the headache we've associated with our migraine disease is considered a primary headache. However, we can develop secondary headaches at any point during our lives related to other organic disorders and comorbid diseases.

So, let's apply this information to our wellness plans. First, we'll take a look at my headache types and comorbid diseases:

- At the time I took responsibility for my health and shifted my focus from illness to wellness, my headache types included migraine with aura, migraine without aura, chronic migraine related to rebound headaches, tension-type headaches, headaches related to a neck injury, and sinus headaches related to episodes of sinusitis.

- The only comorbid disease that bothered me was my mitral valve prolapse, as the disorder exaggerated my sympathetic nervous system response to stress and magnified my headache pain.

Now, it's your turn. If you haven't already done so, grab a pencil and paper and make a list of your headache types and comorbid diseases:

- You may notice that your headache types are different from mine and, for example, may include migraine without aura and chronic tension-type headaches.

- As well, your comorbid diseases may be different and, for example, may include depression and chronic fatigue syndrome.

Already you can see that our wellness plans are going to vary. In the chapters ahead, I will show you how to choose integrative therapies that best suit your needs. For example, if you do not have a neck injury like I do, you may not require physical or chiropractic therapy as part of your plan. However, if you suffer from depression, a moderate exercise program may be just the thing to boost your spirits and relieve your pain.

CHAPTER THREE

Identifying Your Migraine Triggers

ONCE YOU HAVE YOUR diagnosis of migraine disease, you need to know about triggers. Triggers are the stimuli that excite oversensitive neurons and initiate the chain of events that lead to our migraine attacks. In the process, they can irritate cranial nerves, inflame surrounding tissues, promote vascular irregularities, and cause fluctuations in neurotransmitters like serotonin and glutamate.

Although scientific evidence is often insufficient, inconclusive, or debatable, the triggers we look at in this chapter include foods and beverages, environmental factors, hormones, magnesium deficiency, and alterations in our physical and emotional states. And, even though stress is not considered a trigger by many experts in the field, I will address the significant impact of stress on our disease.

That said, the first, and most important, thing I did to reduce the frequency and severity of my migraine attacks was to identify my responsible triggers. The next, and the most difficult thing, because I had to accept my disease and take responsibility for my health, was to manage my identified triggers.

To reduce the frequency and severity of your migraine attacks, it's important to identify your triggers. Although you may find the task difficult in the beginning, your bigger challenge will be to manage your triggers. This is because, like me you're going to have to take responsibility for your own health. In doing so, more than likely, you will have to make substantial changes in what you eat and drink, your eating and drinking habits, your lifestyle, and how you cope with stress. But, before getting to these changes, let's work our way through triggers.

To start with, take a look at some general information about triggers. Triggers may be within our control—for example, what we eat and drink—or uncontrollable—for example, a change in the weather pattern. As well, while one trigger may initiate our migraine attacks, often it takes a combination, or loading, of triggers to precipitate an attack. For instance, one piece of pizza may be okay but, when combined with a larger portion, another food trigger, an alcoholic beverage, a movie with a lot of action and flashing lights, and a fight with our partner, we may be in serious trouble. Also, it might take a couple of hours, several hours, or a few days, for a given trigger to kick in. In addition, it's important to remember that we're individuals. Even though I just gave a global example, the type, number, and combination of triggers necessary to bring on a migraine attack vary with each person. This is where you find out how to become your own expert and policeman.

Food and Beverage Triggers

The most controversial of all our triggers are the foods we ingest and the beverages we drink. But, before you look at these, let me explain the difference between a food allergy and a food sensitivity, or intolerance.

A food allergy produces an immune response in the body that is reflected in symptoms like swelling of the lips and tongue, hives, shortness of breath, closure of the throat, and in some cases anaphylaxis. If you suspect you're allergic to a food, you should see a doctor for a diagnosis.

A migraine attack is usually not related to a food allergy. In most instances, our oversensitive neurons respond to the chemicals and additives in the foods and beverages we ingest. If you have food and beverage sensitivities, the following chemicals and additives are ones you might want to avoid:

Tyramine

- Is a chemical produced during the oxidation or fermentation of protein-rich foods and is found in a whole list of foods, including aged cheeses, bananas, avocados, fava beans, garbanzo beans, lima beans, organ meats like liver, pickled foods, canned soup, nuts, peanut butter, tomatoes, and soy sauce.

- Can cause blood vessels to dilate.

Tannin

- Is a chemical used to clarify wine and beer and is found in a number of foods, including chocolate, cheeses, ice cream, nuts, bananas, smoked foods, and cigarette smoke.

- A diet rich in tannins may affect serotonin levels.

- Many foods containing tannins may also contain tyramine, as just shown, and other amines.

- Tannins may increase sensitivity to other triggers, such as hormonal and environmental stimuli.

Aspartame

- Is an artificial sweetener used in numerous foods and beverages including diet sodas.

- Thought to affect the levels of excitatory neurotransmitters in the brain, including glutamate.

Alcohol

- Is a colorless liquid made from fermentation of sugars and starches.

- Can cause blood vessels to dilate.

- As well, the ethanol has a diuretic effect on the body that can lead to dehydration.

Caffeine

- Is a bitter, white alkaloid present in coffee, tea, sodas, energy drinks, and some foods.

- Can cause blood vessels to constrict, which may abort a migraine; however, it is also a stimulant and a diuretic.

- Excessive use or withdrawal may initiate the chain of events that lead to a migraine attack.

Phenylethylamine

- Is an amino acid that occurs naturally in many proteins and can be extracted for use as a dietary supplement.

- Is found in chocolate.

- Can increase the levels of tyramine in the body.

Sulfites

- Are common preservatives used in foods and are present in fermented beverages and wines.

- Can cause blood vessels to dilate.

Nitrites

- Used to enhance foods and preserve flavor in foods like bacon, ham, pepperoni, and other processed meats.

- Can cause blood vessels to dilate.

Gluten

- Is a type of protein found in wheat, barley, rye, and (to a lesser degree) oats that is difficult to digest. May be added to a number of processed foods as a stabilizer, emulsifier, thickener, starch, or hydrolyzed plant protein.

- Some studies show a correlation between gluten sensitivity, or intolerance, and migraine attacks:

    - Thought that inflammation of the central nervous system and/or malabsorption of vitamins and minerals such as magnesium may precipitate migraine attacks in migraineurs with sensitivity.

    - Other symptoms associated with gluten sensitivity include bloating, diarrhea, fatigue, anemia, nerve pain, balance and gait disorders (ataxia), and seizures.

Monosodium glutamate (MSG)

- Is a sodium salt derived from glutamic acid, an amino acid found naturally in both plant and animal protein, and is added to a number of foods like sauces, gravies, processed meats, packaged foods, and canned soups and vegetables to enhance flavor.

- Studies are inconclusive, but some people report an increase in migraine headaches related to the ingestion of food or beverages that contain MSG:

  - A possible explanation is that the processed glutamic acid in MSG may overexcite brain cells in migraineurs with a sensitivity and precipitate migraine attacks; however, more research is necessary. (See Table 3.1 for a list of ingredients that may trigger migraine attacks in those sensitive to MSG.)

- Other symptoms that may be associated with MSG sensitivity include nausea and vomiting; diarrhea; tingling, numbness, or burning sensation of the face, ears, arms, legs, or feet; chest tightness, rapid or irregular heartbeat; visual disturbances; sensitivity to light; muscle weakness; slurred speech; balance problems; dizziness; lightheadedness; extreme thirst; dry mouth; runny nose; water retention; bloated or swollen abdomen; and a feeling of inebriation (if you're in an environment where alcohol is being served, people may assume you're drunk).

The list of foods and beverages that may contain one or more of these chemicals or additives is exhaustive. I've included some of them with their respective categories. For a more comprehensive list of foods and beverages that may in isolation, combination, or loading trigger your migraine attacks, please see the upcoming "Foods and Beverages" sidebar.

TABLE 3.1: INGREDIENTS THAT MAY TRIGGER MIGRAINE ATTACKS IN THOSE WITH MSG SENSITIVITY

Hydrolyzed protein	Natural flavoring, flavors
Autolyzed yeast, yeast extract, yeast food	Citric acid
	Protease
Glutamic acid, potassium glutamate	Maltodextrin
	Carrageenan
Textured protein	Whey protein
Sodium, or calcium, caseinate	Whey protein concentrate
	Pectin
Anything protein fortified	Soy protein, soy sauce
Anything fermented	Malt extract or flavoring
Anything ultrapasteurized	Anything enzyme modified
Barley malt	Gelatin
Broth, stock	Hydrolyzed oat flour
Bouillon	

You need to be aware that dairy products can increase mucus production, put pressure on your sinus membranes, and magnify the sinus component of your migraines. Hot and spicy foods can increase the heat in your body, lead to vasodilation, and trigger an attack. As well, some reports indicate that a diet high in fats can trigger migraine attacks. For more information on cooling, warming, and neutral foods, please refer to Chapter Eight.

Foods and Beverages That May in Isolation, Combination, or Loading Trigger Migraine Attacks

Aged and unpasteurized cheeses including Parmesan, cheddar (most yellow cheeses), blue cheese (Stilton, Roquefort, Gorgonzola), Brie, Camembert, Monterey Jack, mozzarella, and Gruyere

continued

Avocados

Bananas

Beans including lima, broad, Italian, navy, pinto, and garbanzo

Beer and spirits

Berry pie filling, or canned berries

Brewer's yeast including sourdough bread, yeast breads straight from oven, yeast coffee cake, donuts, pizza dough, and soft pretzels

Cabbage, sauerkraut

Canned soups, instant soups, and noodles

Chicken liver and other organ meats

Chili peppers, onions

Chocolate

Citrus fruit (grapefruit, oranges)

Cocoa, cola drinks, tea and coffee

Corn syrup

Diet drinks

Eggs

Fatty and fried foods

Flavored potato and taco chips

Gravies, dips, sauces, seasoning, and sauce mixes, ketchup, mayonnaise, steak sauce, vinegar (except white)

Lentils

Licorice

Many salad dressings

Meat tenderizer

Most fast foods

Nuts including peanuts, pistachios, cashews, and almonds; peanut butter

Packaged foods such as pasta and meat combinations, and cake and muffin mixes

Pickled, preserved, or marinated foods such as olives and pickles

Pineapple, papaya, passion fruit

Processed, smoked, cured, or pickled meat or fish, including most deli meats, ham, bacon, hot dogs, salami, pepperoni, smoked salmon, pickled herring

Red meat, pork

Red plums, prunes, raisins, figs, and dried fruits

Red wine (white wine may be tolerated in moderation)

Seafood such as salmon and shellfish

Seasoned salt

Seeds, including pumpkin and sunflower

Snow peas

Soy sauce, miso, tempeh

Spinach

Strawberries

Tomatoes, tomato sauce, tomato paste

Wheat

Yogurt, buttermilk, sour cream, whole milk, and ice cream

How to Identify and Manage Your Food and Beverage Triggers

The relationship of food and beverage triggers to migraine attacks can be complicated. You may find that very few of the foods and beverages listed in the "Foods and Beverages" sidebar give you a migraine attack, or you might have a sensitivity to so many that you cannot identify specific ones.

To make matters a little more confusing, a reaction to what you eat or drink usually occurs within a few hours after ingestion. However, a reaction to MSG can be immediate or as late as forty-eight hours after consumption. Also, eating a product once a week may not cause a reaction, but eating products two or three days in a row might (cumulative). In addition, a reaction may be more severe if you accompany the food with an alcoholic beverage. As well, it may not be what you consume that gives you the migraine attack, but when and how much you eat or drink. For example, dehydration and hypoglycemia can trigger a migraine attack. Thus not drinking enough water, fasting, and skipped or delayed meals can have a significant impact on the frequency and severity of your attacks.

So, now to help you out. Some sources recommend an elimination diet. However, given the number of food and beverage triggers, and the fact that they vary with each person, a more reasonable approach is to keep a food diary, or calendar. I prefer a calendar and tell you why later in this chapter.

Whichever method you select, you should record all the foods and beverages you consume each day, along with the approximate times you ate or drank, and any migraine symptoms you experienced. Any food triggers you identify should be avoided. It might be helpful to have your doctor, a dietitian, or nutritionist guide you through the process to help you avoid any nutritional deficits and to recommend appropriate supplements.

Some general guidelines I've incorporated into my wellness plan (many of these were given to me by Dr. Mao during my first visit and can be found in his book, *Secrets of Self-Healing*

(Avery, 2008) and that you may want to include in your wellness plan are

- Read labels. You may spend an extra long time in the market in the beginning, but the results will be worth the time you sacrifice.

- Avoid processed or packaged foods with artificial colors, flavors, additives, chemicals, or preservatives.

- If you think you're gluten sensitive (refer to symptoms mentioned earlier), avoid foods that contain gluten.

- If you think you're MSG sensitive (refer to symptoms mentioned earlier), avoid foods that contain MSG (see Table 3.1 for a list of ingredients that may trigger your migraine attacks if you're MSG sensitive).

- Avoid fast food. If I'm going to be away from home over a lunch or dinner hour and I'm traveling by air or car and have no idea what, if anything, I'll be served or where I can find something suitable to eat, I pack a sandwich.

- Eat wholesome, organic foods (United States Department of Agriculture or USDA approved) with no antibiotics, growth hormones, pesticides, additives, preservatives, artificial colors or flavorings. If organic fruits and vegetables are too expensive or difficult for you to obtain, whenever possible, substitute natural foods and beverages that are minimally processed and have no artificial ingredients, added colors, chemicals, or preservatives. Thoroughly wash non-organic fruits and vegetables in salt water or with a vegetable and fruit wash to remove chemicals and pesticides.

- Avoiding your triggers, eat a variety of fresh fruits, vegetables, whole grains, beans, legumes, fish, and poultry to help prevent fluctuations in your serotonin levels. (Foods do not contain serotonin, but certain foods, for example pasta, candy, cereal, and a number of other refined carbohydrates and sugars, can stimulate the release of serotonin. The effects can last up to two or three hours, then wear off, and your serotonin levels drop.)

- Avoiding your triggers, favor fiber-rich foods such as leafy green vegetables, parsley, onions, brown rice, bran, carrots, celery, asparagus, papaya, pineapple, cherries, grapes, prunes, and fresh herbs and spices such as ginger, oregano, rosemary, cilantro, dill, sage, mint, and turmeric to help with digestion and elimination.

- Avoid spicy foods (as mentioned earlier).

- Avoid starchy, rich, and greasy foods (as mentioned).

- Avoid dairy products (as mentioned).

- Avoid chocolate and caffeine. Initially, these stimulants can increase your serotonin levels. However, when consumed in large quantities, over time they can deplete your serotonin levels (controversial, but some sources say infrequent, small amounts of these substances may be okay).

- Avoid alcohol and red wine (small amounts of white wine may be okay). Not only does alcohol cause vasodilation and fluctuations in your serotonin levels, it is also dehydrating. If you're going to drink, the guideline for the general public is one glass of water for every glass of alcohol consumed. However, given the sensitivity of our neurons to stimulants, don't be surprised if this doesn't work for you.

- Drink a minimum of eight to ten glasses of water a day (dehydration can trigger your migraine attack).

- Eat small, regular meals at a table and try to have your breakfast before 9 a.m., lunch before 1 p.m., and dinner before 7 p.m. (skipped meals, fasting, and dieting can cause hypoglycemia and trigger your migraine attack).

- Don't eat late at night, and don't lie down immediately after eating (can interfere with your sleep pattern, cause fatigue, and stimulate your migraine attack).

- If you're eating at a restaurant, check with the chef (not the waiter or waitress) if you're concerned about food allergies or sensitivities. My husband has become accustomed to letting the chef know that I'm extremely sensitive to additives, in particular MSG, and that the restaurant might want to call the local paramedics if I'm exposed to any harmful ingredients.

- If you're dining at family or friends' homes, don't be afraid to relate any food allergies or sensitivities you may have. It's nice to do this beforehand, but if you don't have that chance, offending the host or hostess is less of a price to pay than the migraine attack that is likely to follow.

- If a meal is going to be served later than your normal dining hour, or you're not certain if the food will be appropriate for you, eat a healthy snack before you go.

At this point, it's important for you to note that once you have your migraine attacks under control, you may be able to add back in some of the foods you have eliminated. However, begin with small portions. And remember, everything in moderation, and watch out for combinations. For instance, since I had been migraine free for many months, I dropped my guard. I was at a dinner gathering where a number of courses were served, many of which contained an assortment of cheeses and red meat. The extreme thirst, rapid and irregular heart rate, muscle weakness, headache, nausea, and vomiting I experienced a few hours later were unpleasant, but worthwhile reminders that I'm still vulnerable.

Environmental Triggers

Because our migraine brains are more excitable than others, our attacks may be precipitated by anything that irritates our cranial nerves. The most common environmental triggers that drive our neurons crazy include

- Bright lights including sunlight, computer glare, fluorescent and flickering lights

- Loud noises

- Strong smells such as perfume, cologne, gasoline, cleaning products, pesticides, paint, cigarette smoke, and smoke from wood-burning stoves and fireplaces

- Weather changes, including significant fluctuations in temperature and humidity, overcast skies

- Altitude and barometric pressure changes (thought that blood vessels may contract and expand in response to alterations in oxygen levels)

How to Identify and Manage Your Environmental Triggers

When I first visited the migraine clinic, I was plagued by every environmental trigger I've mentioned. For example, whenever my husband and I travelled by land, sea, or air, I would get a sharp, stabbing pain in my head, followed by a tremendous, throbbing migraine headache. I could actually feel the pressure in my head increase. Smoke is another instant trigger for me. Immediately my sinuses fill up with pressure that radiates to the back of my neck and then explodes into a migraine headache. Bright lights are another pain for me. My vision starts to blur, and sometimes within minutes, I can feel a throbbing at my temples.

At the migraine clinic, both the psychologist and the biofeedback therapist told me that if I learned to control my insides, the outside would take care of itself. I was dubious, but nevertheless, every week I sat in a recliner chair for at least an hour and listened to a tape of waves rolling onto shore while I belly-breathed, meditated, and envisioned the blood flowing from my swollen brain to the constricted vessels of my hands and feet (see Chapters Eight and Nine for more details on deep-breathing techniques, biofeedback therapy, and meditation).

Then, after several visits with Dr. Mao, numerous acupuncture treatments that I continue every six weeks, more instruction and practice with deep breathing and relaxation techniques, and meditation, I discovered that these guys were right. Knowing how to calm myself and balance my insides has enabled me to desensitize my body's response to external stimuli, without using OTC and prescription medications.

Now each day, I spend at least an hour (usually in the early afternoon), sitting or lying comfortably where I clear my mind, relax, deep breathe, and meditate. Often, I fall into a short, but deep, healing sleep. Some of the other things I've incorporated into my wellness plan to make myself as migraine-free as possible, and that you may want to as well, include

- Always wear a hat and sunglasses in bright sunlight (ten minutes in a hot sun without a hat, and my head begins to throb).

- Where possible, minimize your time driving at night.

- Use lamps or overhead fixtures that provide soft light. If necessary, wear your sunglasses in markets, department stores, or other environments where fluorescent or bright lights are beyond your control.

- Take frequent breaks from your computer and television.

- Turn the volume down on whatever the source of your music.

- Wear earplugs in noisy environments beyond your control.

- If you smoke, stop. Today it is much easier to avoid smoke-filled settings as many public places are smoke free. However, if you have family or friends who still smoke, then ask them to smoke outside. If you want to join them for a visit, stay upwind.

- If wood-burning stoves or fireplaces bother you, convert to gas, or electric, if possible.

- Control other smells such as perfumes, cologne, cleaning supplies, pesticides, and paint in your home by using products that are less problematic (in environments beyond your control, avoid when possible).

- Stay hydrated when flying, hiking, traveling long distances by car, and while on vacation (changes in temperature, weather, and altitude are thought to cause changes in blood vessels in response to oxygen demand).

- Drink plenty of water and avoid exercise the first few days after a change to a higher altitude.

- Avoid hot tubs, saunas, and extremely hot baths and showers, especially when combined with ingestion of any type of alcohol (can cause your blood vessels to dilate).

Hormonal Migraine Triggers

Fluctuations in the levels of estrogen and progesterone are thought to be triggers for migraine attacks in about sixty to seventy percent of women, particularly those of child-bearing age. If you suffer from hormonal migraine attacks, you might want to know that all women don't respond to fluctuations in estrogen and progesterone in the same way.

Some women may be more sensitive to changes prior to the onset of their menstrual cycle, others during their menstrual cycle, others during pregnancy, and still others at the onset of menopause when hormones really shift. As well, birth control pills and pregnancy can affect the frequency and severity of attacks for some women and decrease them for others. Let's take a closer look at these variations:

Menstruation

- True menstrual migraine occurs during your menstrual period. These attacks are without aura. You may have attacks with aura at other times during the month related to other triggers and chronic migraine.

- Menstrual-related migraine (MRM) occurs two days before to three days after the onset of menstruation. Attacks may occur at other times during the menstrual cycle such as ovulation. Like true menstrual migraine, these attacks are believed to be without aura.

Oral contraceptives

- May accentuate the fluctuation of your hormones and increase the frequency, duration, and severity of your migraine attacks.

- May be the initial onset of your migraine attacks.

Pregnancy

- May increase the frequency, duration, and severity of your migraine attacks.

- Your migraine attacks may decrease.

- May be the initial onset of your migraine attacks.

Hormone replacement therapy (HRT)

- May increase your migraine attacks, especially if your dose is cyclical (for example: five days on, two days off).

Menopause

- Your migraine attacks may increase in frequency, duration, and severity.

- Your migraine attacks may resolve.

- May be the initial onset of your migraine attacks.

How to Identify and Manage Your Hormonal Triggers

Like any other type of migraine, keeping track of your migraine attacks with a journal or calendar will help you identify the pattern of your hormonal migraines. I mentioned earlier that I prefer a calendar. This is because migraine triggers can overlap. For example, the foods and beverages you crave when you're hormonal can also trigger or exacerbate your attacks.

To manage your hormonal migraine attacks, it's helpful for you to understand how fluctuations in the levels of your hormones can affect the neurotransmitters in your brain. In particular, when estrogen levels rise, there is a corresponding increase in serotonin levels. When there is a drop in estrogen levels, serotonin levels decrease. And, if you recall, as I mentioned in Chapter One, the neurotransmitters dopamine and norepinephrine tend to fluctuate with serotonin levels.

This relationship between estrogen and these neurotransmitters may be responsible for many of the mood swings you experience during your menstrual cycle, pregnancy, or menopause. For example, low levels of estrogen and serotonin may cause you to feel depressed, anxious, or irritable. High levels of estrogen and serotonin are mood elevators and may make you feel calm, full, happy, and relaxed.

Low levels of serotonin may also explain many of the food cravings you experience as your hormones fluctuate. As well, since serotonin enhances endorphins (our natural pain-killers), low levels of the neurotransmitter may be why some women claim their hormone-related migraine headaches are more intense than their other ones.

Keeping these things in mind, some suggestions to reduce the number and severity of your hormonal attacks include

- Keep track of your monthly cycle and record any migraine attacks and associated symptoms.

- Take extra steps to reduce all the other triggers we have, or will, address in this chapter. I will repeat this many times throughout the book. A healthy diet that avoids or eliminates your personal triggers as well as simple carbohydrates, refined sugars, processed foods, and those loaded with chemicals and preservatives can be one of your biggest allies against this disease (refer to food and beverage triggers).

- Learn how to manage stress (for more on stress, see the upcoming section "A Word About Stress and Migraine Disease"), as stress can deplete your hormones and increase the frequency and severity of your attacks. You will find that the ability to manage the stress in your life will be another major ally in your battle with this disease.

- If you're on a birth control pill and your attacks increase, see your doctor about changing to an alternative method of contraception.

- If you're on cyclical hormone replacement therapy and your attacks increase, ask your doctor about a low-dose, continuous therapy. (I went through surgical menopause when I was forty-one years old. With cyclical therapy—five days on, two days off—my migraine attacks worsened. When I switched to a low-dose hormone every day, they improved.)

- Many sources recommend magnesium and/or progesterone replacement therapy (check with your doctor and see if such treatments are appropriate for you).

- NSAIDs (nonsteroidal anti-inflammatory drugs) and other migraine medications may be helpful. See your doctor for those that will provide the most effective relief for your type of hormonal migraine attack (see Chapter Four for more information about medications).

- Herbs like feverfew and butterbur may be helpful (see Chapter Eight for more information about herbs).

- If you're pregnant or trying to conceive, consult with your obstetrician or other healthcare practitioner before taking any supplement, drug, or herb.

At this point, it's important to note that lower levels of cortisol (see the section on stress later in this chapter) and testosterone can increase the frequency of migraine attacks and cluster headaches in men (refer to the "International Headache Society Classification of Headaches" section in Chapter Two). As well, some reports indicate low levels of testosterone can contribute to the frequency of migraine attacks in women who have had their ovaries removed or have reached menopause. A blood test can determine if you're deficient in testosterone and need replacement therapy.

One final thing to be aware of is that sexual intercourse can either abort or precipitate a migraine attack for some people. Avoiding stimulants, such as alcohol, prior to sex may help prevent orgasm migraines. If the problem is a new onset or your headache changes character in any way, a visit to your doctor is in order to rule out an underlying disorder.

Magnesium Deficiency

Magnesium is a mineral in our bodies that is important for a number of functions, including protein synthesis, neuromuscular function, regulation of nerve cells, and vessel tone (keeps your blood vessels from going into spasm). As well, magnesium is believed to be involved with the regulation of serotonin.

Low levels of magnesium can precipitate the chain of events that lead to our migraine attacks. They are often associated with other migraine triggers such as alcohol and caffeine (deplete magnesium from our body) and menstruation (levels drop right before the onset of your period). In addition, conditions comorbid to migraine disease such as mitral valve prolapse, anxiety disorders, and epilepsy may exhibit magnesium deficiency.

How to Identify and Manage Magnesium Deficiency

As mentioned in the preceding discussion, numerous things are associated with magnesium deficiency, including menstruation, alcohol, caffeine, and a diet lacking in magnesium. Magnesium is found in whole, unprocessed foods such as green leafy vegetables, nuts, wheat germ, bananas, soy products, milk, and unrefined grains (again, caution as some of these may be a migraine trigger for you).

Reports are controversial, but some research suggests that we may have lower blood levels of magnesium than people who don't have migraines. Symptoms of magnesium deficiency include irritability, agitation, anxiety, confusion, insomnia, restless leg syndrome, muscle spasms, twitching, seizures, weakness, poor coordination, nausea and vomiting, irregular heartbeat, and rapid heart rate. If you suspect that you're magnesium deficient, check with your doctor. A simple blood test will determine your blood level.

Your doctor, or other health professional, is the one to suggest a supplement or replacement therapy as there are many different types of magnesium and too much magnesium can cause harmful side effects. Also, there are many medications that you might be taking that can interfere with blood levels of magnesium such as diuretics, some antibiotics, calcium channel blockers and other blood pressure medications, chemotherapy drugs, steroids, hormone replacement therapy, and digoxin. Side effects of too much magnesium include upset stomach and diarrhea, nausea and vomiting, hypotension (low blood pressure), flushing, slow heart rate, lethargy, drowsiness, and even death.

A word of caution: If you're a renal patient, you must be careful with magnesium intake as you are unable to excrete excessive amounts of the mineral via your kidneys.

Physical and Emotional Triggers

Physical and emotional triggers that may set off migraine attacks include, but are not limited to the following:

- Anger (clenched teeth)

- Arguments (see muscle tension)

- Break in routine (especially on weekends, holidays, and vacations)

- Change in sleep patterns (oversleeping, disrupted, not enough)

- Crying due to sadness, depression

- Dehydration, especially on hot days and with exercise

- Dieting, fasting (hypoglycemia as mentioned earlier)

- Drugs including marijuana, amphetamines, and cocaine

- Excessive exercise

- Fatigue, chronic fatigue

- Illness such as viral infections, colds, flu, allergies

- Lack of sleep, sleep deprivation

- Muscle tension in the scalp, jaw, neck, shoulders, upper back (more common in tension-type headache)

- Nightmares, traumatic dreams (clenched teeth and muscle tension)

- Poor posture (more common in tension-type headache; tension-type headache may coexist with migraine)

- Skipped, delayed, or inadequate meals (hypoglycemia as mentioned earlier)

- Withdrawal from caffeine, alcohol, drugs

How to Identify and Manage Physical and Emotional Triggers

Many of our physical and emotional triggers can be provoked by stressful situations (see the next section). For example, in my case, many times while studying for exams or preparing for an important lecture or seminar, I didn't eat regular meals (if I ate at all), slept poorly while I rehashed study questions or lecture notes all night, and consequently woke with a tremendous headache and nausea.

Besides daily biofeedback techniques, relaxation exercises, and meditation, some general guidelines to reduce physical and emotional triggers I've found helpful, and you may as well, include

- Keep a regular meal schedule. If your stomach is in knots because of a stressful situation and you cannot swallow a bite of food, calm yourself down through breathing and relaxation techniques and meditation (remember, the stress response slows the movement of food through your intestines). When you're ready (you may feel your stomach growl), drink a nutritious shake or smoothie, or eat a small portion of food.

- If you have house guests, or are a house guest, and your normal meal schedule is in jeopardy, compromise (my worst is brunch as I have to eat breakfast). Eat at your regular time and keep them company at theirs.

- Avoid dieting and fasting (if you want to lose weight, eat smaller portions and pick up your exercise).

- If you haven't done so already, check with your physician and then begin a daily regimen of cardiovascular and stretching exercises. Low to moderate intensity exercises, such as walking and sports that rely on endurance rather than power like swimming, hiking, long-distance running, tai chi exercises and yoga, can increase your serotonin levels.

- As I've mentioned numerous times, drink plenty of water.

- If you're cutting back on caffeine, alcohol, or other stimulants, minimize other triggers to reduce the severity of an expected attack.

- If, like I do, you have a set time for meditation and you have company or are visiting family or friends, don't be afraid to dismiss yourself from their presence and claim your much-needed healing time.

- Keep a regular sleep schedule (oversleeping on weekends, holidays, and vacation can precipitate a migraine). If you have house guests or are a house guest and their bedtime is later than yours, don't be bashful about excusing yourself for the evening. Likewise, arise at your normal hour and be prepared to make yourself breakfast.

- If you have trouble sleeping or are bothered by interrupted sleep, indulge in a session of self-gratification such as a warm bath or a cup of soothing herbal tea before bedtime (avoid anything that might stimulate your mind including television, phone conversations, and reading materials).

- Sit up straight. Muscle tension in the shoulders, upper back, head, and neck irritates the cranial nerves. (Since my neck injury, I've become acutely aware of poor posture.)

- If you feel an attack coming on, avoid extreme exercise (a short, leisurely walk may help increase your serotonin levels and abort the attack).

- Remember, you have the ability to control how you respond to stressful situations (see the next section). When you're performing under continuous pressure, your body's natural defenses break down. You become susceptible to illnesses like colds, flu, and allergies, which themselves can precipitate a migraine attack.

- If arguments and emotions such as anger have you clenching your teeth and tightening the muscles in your face head and neck, find a way to express your anger in a healthy fashion (see Chapter Seven for more information on emotional balancing).

- Crying can be a good way to release stress; however it may cause muscle tightness and tension in the body. Deep breathing and neck and shoulder stretches may help prevent the onset of a headache.

A Word About Stress and Migraine Disease

Since many of the integrative therapies I talk about in Parts Two and Three affect the sympathetic and parasympathetic nervous systems, it's crucial that you understand what happens to our bodies and our emotions when we're stressed. To begin with, let's look at some general information about stress.

Stress is the normal physiological response of our bodies to any demand or change. When we perceive a threat, our nervous system responds by releasing a flood of hormones, including but not limited to epinephrine (adrenalin), norepinephrine (noradrenalin), and cortisol. Our heart rate, blood pressure, and respiration increase, our muscles tighten, and almost all of our other body systems, including our immune system, digestive system, and sensory organs, gear up to fight our challenger (see Chapter One for more information about the nervous system).

Stress can be related to environmental, chemical, physical, or emotional challenges. It's important for you to be aware that our bodies don't distinguish between these threats. Our bodies react the same way whether we're overcome with noise at a rock concert, we're inhaling toxic fumes at a chemical spill, we're exposed to an immediate danger like a fire, we have a life-threatening illness such as cancer, we're the victim of a traumatic injury, we're anxious about an exam or job interview, or we're worried about a teenager who hasn't come home by curfew or troublesome bills we cannot pay.

Some stress can be good for us. Acute stress (short-term), or good stress, is short-lived and is our body's way of helping us get through a crisis—for example, the momentum to flee a burning building, finish a term paper, or tackle a new job. It keeps us on our toes and allows us to stay focused, energetic, and alert. In this stage, levels of adrenalin, noradrenalin, and cortisol are high, giving us the energy to respond to the challenge at hand. We may feel wired, excited, and have an abundance of physical strength. Once the emergency has passed, the levels of these hormones return to normal.

Chronic stress (long-term), or bad stress, is long-lived and not good for us. Some examples include continued exposure to chemicals and pollution, hectic lifestyles, jobs that challenge our physical and emotional capabilities, persistent unemployment, not knowing how to relax or manage our time, worrying about things beyond our control or that we cannot fix in the middle of the night, and long-term illnesses.

In these instances, levels of adrenalin, noradrenalin, and cortisol begin to drop and may become depleted. Levels of DHEA (dehydroepiandrosterone), a steroid produced by the adrenal glands and used to make estrogen and testosterone, start to fall, and neurotransmitters like serotonin are affected. Our body's metabolism slows down and we may feel tired, fatigued, and gain weight, especially around the middle. A decrease in our sex hormones can cause hormonal imbalances and loss of libido (sex drive), while low levels of serotonin can lead to emotional disturbances like anxiety and depression.

Now, let's apply this information to migraine disease. There are a number of ways stress can provoke or aggravate migraine attacks in those of us who have the disease. However, because an individual's perception of stress varies (what stresses me may not stress you), you need to be aware that the International Headache Society has removed stress from the list of triggers associated with migraine disease. Stress is, though, recognized as a trigger for tension-type headaches and acknowledged as a factor that makes us more susceptible to our triggers—for example, physical and emotional triggers (as previously discussed).

As well, stress is recognized as a factor that can magnify the duration and intensity of migraine attacks—for example, hormonal migraines (as discussed)—and if prolonged is thought to increase the frequency of migraine attacks and lead to the development of chronic migraines. Also, you need to know that a migraine attack itself can stimulate the sympathetic nervous system and initiate the stress response just discussed. In addition, the relaxation phase following an episode of stress can precipitate a migraine attack known as a *let down migraine.*

Although stress may be difficult for us to avoid, the good news is that we can take measures to limit our exposure and calm our body's reaction to the persistent stimuli. Some of these interventions include switching to a healthy diet, avoiding stimulants, learning how to manage our time, and taking time to introduce stress reduction techniques like biofeedback and exercise (already discussed in this chapter) into our lifestyle. In the chapters ahead, I will share a number of other treatments and therapies, such as acupuncture, meditation, mind-body exercises, and energy healing techniques, that can promote relaxation, help stabilize your serotonin levels, increase your endorphins, and decrease the frequency and severity of your attacks.

Looking Back and Glimpsing Ahead

In this chapter, you found out what triggers are and how to identify some of the ones that initiate your migraine attacks. As well, you discovered a number of ways to manage your triggers and reduce the frequency and severity of your attacks. You also learned about stress and the impact it has on our disease.

Now, apply this information to our wellness plans. I've met many people who have no idea how to identify their triggers. As I stated earlier, the task can be difficult. So, examine how I learned to identify my triggers:

- To begin with, I began to keep a monthly calendar (the kind with big squares to write in, and you can see overlapping triggers at a glance).

- I recorded every possible trigger for at least three days prior to a headache. For example, I wrote down everything I had to eat and drink; documented sudden changes in the weather (humidity, overhead mist, and thunder storms, in particular) and interruptions in my daily routine and sleep patterns (whether I was traveling or had visitors whose requests interfered with my schedule); and noted bright lights like sunlight off the water when we spent time at the beach or off white snow when we were skiing, loud noises such as rock music on high volume, and annoying odors such as cigarette smoke.

- Then I watched for a pattern. For example, I noticed that if I ate dairy products when it was overcast or raining, I got a migraine headache. Other times, they didn't affect me. If I ate chocolate or anything that had chocolate in it like a rich dessert, I had a problem. It seemed every time my husband and I went out to dinner or attended events like weddings, birthdays, and even funerals, I got a migraine. Except for a glass or two of white wine, alcohol was a definite "no." Always my migraine attacks were worse in the presence of large crowds, loud music, and bright lights.

Once I identified my triggers, the challenge began. To manage my triggers, I began by eliminating or, where possible, avoiding the ones that seemed most problematic. To help myself out, I focused on the suggestions and guidelines I've shared with you throughout this chapter.

As I tossed my triggers aside, I began to document my progress to recovery. On the same calendar I used to identify my triggers, I recorded what measures I took to abort the pain. For example, was medication required, or was I able to abort the attack with the incorporation of integrative therapies like ice packs on my forehead and the base of my neck? I had started acupuncture and kept track of my appointments, and as I incorporated more stress reduction and healing techniques into my wellness plan, I added them in.

Soon my calendar was packed. But a strange thing began to happen. My migraine attacks became less and less, and the nausea and vomiting, which had been so horrific for me, began to disappear. Even more enlightening, I watched my dependence on Imitrex (changed by Dr. B. to Relpax, a newer triptan) drop from daily to once a week, then to once a month, then to once a year, and now to a supply I keep in the refrigerator for emergencies, but rarely have to use.

To top things off, the events and occasions that I'd previously had to miss, because I was in bed with a headache, took over the spots my migraine attacks left vacant. I had my life back! I can't tell you how great that feels.

Now, it's your turn. If you haven't already done so, decide whether you want to keep a journal or a calendar and follow my guidelines as you proceed through the months ahead:

- Write down your triggers as I just described. If you have hormonal migraine attacks, include these on the appropriate dates.

- You will notice that your triggers will differ from mine (remember we're unique in what sets us off).

- As well, the measures you take to manage your triggers will evolve as you learn more about stress reduction therapies and techniques and are able to pick and choose the ones that work best for you.

It will take you time, but as a pattern emerges, you will find that you become your own expert about your triggers and that you will be happy to take on the role of policeman for their management. The more committed you are, the less you will require medication, and the more you will be able to spend time with your family, miss fewer days at work, and enjoy your quality of life.

At this point, you might be thinking, "Isn't a healthy diet, avoiding stimulants, and learning how to manage stress good for everyone?" You are right. Many of the triggers we looked at in this chapter are risk factors for disorders like hypertension, stroke, heart disease, and type 2 diabetes. As well, many of the food triggers, like rich and fatty ones, can lead to obesity when consumed in large quantities. So, look at it this way. The more you stick to your wellness plan, the fewer migraine attacks you'll suffer *and* the lower your risk factors for a number of diseases will be—and in the process, you may even lose or stabilize your weight.

CHAPTER FOUR

How Doctors Determine Which Medication You Should Take

In Chapter Two, we looked at the importance of consulting a physician for a correct diagnosis of our headaches. At that time, after a thorough history and physical examination, your doctor should determine a treatment program for you based on:

- The onset of your migraine attack (for example, is it sudden or gradual).

- The severity of your attacks (for example, is your pain mild or crippling).

- The frequency of your migraine attacks (for example, do they occur once or twice a week, less often, or more often).

- Your symptoms (for example, do you have associated nausea and vomiting that make it difficult for you to take oral medications).

- Coexisting medical conditions or allergies that contraindicate the use of a particular drug (for example, I have a cutaneous form of porphyria that causes me to blister from medications such as barbiturates, antihistamines, antidepressants, and anticonvulsants).

- Any OTC and prescription medications you're taking, as well as herbs and supplements, because they could interfere with the medications your doctor may prescribe (for example, I take many herbs prescribed by Dr. Mao, and Dr. B. is well aware of them).

- The impact of medication on your work and home environment (for example, is drowsiness a factor).

Medications Your Doctor Might Prescribe

Depending on the information you share, your doctor may recommend an OTC drug or prescribe a medication from one or more of the following categories: analgesics, antiemetics, abortive medications, and prophylactic (preventative) drugs. Let's look at some general information about these drugs.

Analgesics are drugs used to control pain. Some analgesics are combined with another drug such as a barbiturate or caffeine to increase the effect of the primary medication. These are known as *combination drugs*.

An antiemetic is a drug used to control our nausea and vomiting. Abortive medications are used to stop headaches at the onset. And a prophylactic drug is used to prevent our migraine attacks.

Routes of administration for these medications that may be helpful for you to understand, include

- **Pills or capsules:** These are absorbed through your gastrointestinal tract, so they are not the best choice if you suffer from nausea and vomiting or delayed gastric emptying. Sublingual forms are held under your tongue until they're dissolved. They are absorbed through the membrane lining your mouth; therefore, they are quick to act.

- **Nasal sprays:** These are absorbed through the membrane lining your nose. They are fast to act, so they are good if your migraine attacks come on suddenly. However, they can leave a bad taste in your mouth. They are an option if you suffer from severe nausea and vomiting and are unable to retain anything you swallow. They are not the best choice if you have a cold or suffer from nasal allergies.

- **Suppositories:** These are absorbed through the membrane of your rectum. Like nasal sprays, they are an option if you cannot retain oral medications. They are not the best choice if you have diarrhea with your migraine attacks.

- **Injections:** These are the most effective if your attacks are rapid and severe. Many people, me included, do not like to self-inject.

- **Patches:** A patch is placed on the skin to deliver a specific dose of the drug through the skin into the bloodstream. An option if nausea and vomiting is so bad that you cannot swallow a pill.

Like our triggers, you need to know that each of us reacts differently to different drugs. So, even though I focus on actions, possible side effects, and contraindications of drugs that may be prescribed for you, I encourage you to read the pharmacy notes and packet inserts on all of your medications. This is your responsibility as well as your doctor's.

As well, because of the danger associated with drug interactions, you should not take any OTC or other drugs, including herbs and supplements, without your doctor's consent. Also, you need to know that your doctor will give you the appropriate dose for each medication prescribed. If you're taking OTC medications, you should not exceed the doses recommended on the label. Taking any of the majority of these medications too frequently or exceeding the recommended doses can cause you to have rebound headaches (see Chapter Two for more information about rebound headaches).

Finally, it's important for you to tell your doctor if you're pregnant or thinking of becoming pregnant. Many of the medications discussed in this chapter can harm your fetus.

So, now let's examine specific medications within each category.

Analgesics

If your migraine attacks are infrequent and you describe your pain as mild to moderate, your doctor may recommend one or more of the following analgesics:

Acetaminophen (Tylenol): This is a pain and fever reducer and has the following properties:

- May work for moderate pain and is most effective if you take it within fifteen minutes of the onset of your headache.

- Has little anti-inflammatory action.

- Does not affect blood-clotting like aspirin and NSAIDs; however, it may affect clotting times if you take it with Coumadin (warfarin).

- Cold, allergy, or sleep medications may contain acetaminophen (may be abbreviated as "APAP") and when taken with Tylenol can cause you to have too much.

- Do not take this drug if you have a history of alcoholism or liver disease, as it will increase the risk of damage to your liver.

Aspirin (Acetylsalicylic Acid–ASA): This is an analgesic, a fever-reducer, and an anti-inflammatory agent (non-steroidal).

- Some reports indicate that 1000 mg of aspirin when taken at the onset of your pain may be equally effective as abortive drugs like sumatriptan.

- Slows the rate of blood clotting, so although it may be helpful in the prevention of heart attacks and strokes in high risk patients, it should not be taken in situations where bleeding might be increased, such as surgeries, dental extractions, gastric irritation or ulcers and if you use blood thinners like Coumadin, without the consent of your doctor.

- May cause hearing problems like ringing in your ears or temporary loss of hearing.

Non-steroidal anti-inflammatory drugs (NSAIDs) such as naproxen, Advil (Advil Migraine), ibuprofen, and Motrin (Motrin Migraine):

- They block the release of prostaglandins, which are chemicals that enhance the sensitivity of pain endings and stimulate the release of inflammatory agents (see Chapter One). Prostaglandins protect the lining of the stomach, so blocking them may result in gastric irritation and cause complications such as stomach pain, heartburn, and bleeding.

- Do not take them without consulting your doctor if you have high blood pressure, kidney, liver, or heart disease, have more than three alcoholic drinks per day, or if you're taking blood thinners such as aspirin or Coumadin.

Narcotic (Opioid) analgesics such as codeine, morphine, Demerol (meperidine), methadone (Dolophine), butorphanol (Stadol NS), Dilaudid (hydromorphone), hydrocodone (Vicotin), oxycodone (OxyContin), and oxymorphone (Numorphan):

- These are narcotic pain relievers that act on the CNS (central nervous system).

- Narcotic analgesics should be prescribed only by your doctor, or an emergency room physician for immediate management of an acute (severe, or breakthrough, migraine attack), when all other interventions are ineffective.

- Disorders such as head injuries; seizures, asthma, or any other chronic lung disease; hypothyroidism; Addison's disease, which is a disease of the adrenal glands; colitis; enlarged prostrate; and drug or alcohol abuse may impact the use of these analgesics.

- Some of these analgesics may be mixed with other medications in a combination migraine drug (see combination migraine medications) to allow a lower dose of the narcotic to be given to relieve pain.

- May make gastrointestinal symptoms, like nausea and vomiting, associated with your migraine attack worse.

- May cause side effects such as drowsiness, confusion, hallucinations, weakness, slow or shallow breathing (respiratory depression), dry mouth, difficulty with urination, and constipation.

- If you use these drugs over a long period of time, you may become physically or mentally dependent.

A word of caution: It's essential that you tell your doctor, or emergency room physician, if you're taking any of the medications in the upcoming "Drugs That May Interact" sidebar, as your doctor needs to control the dosages; otherwise, serious and often life-threatening drug interactions may occur.

At this point, I ought to mention that if you haven't already done so, you should make a list of all your medical diagnoses and what medications you take for each disease. You should carry this list in your wallet, plus have a copy posted on your refrigerator at home in case of a medical emergency where you cannot speak for yourself. In addition, dependent on your diagnoses and the number of drugs you take, you may want to wear a medical alert bracelet or necklace.

Drugs That May Interact with Narcotic Analgesics

CNS depressants: When combined with narcotics, these drugs can intensify your risk for respiratory depression, hypotension, coma, accidental overdose, and death. This category includes

- Alcohol

- Antihistamines such as diphenhydramine or other medications for allergies, hay fever, and colds

- Other prescription pain relievers

- Sedatives, tranquilizers or sleeping pills such as Valium (diazepam), Xanax (alprazolam), and Librium (chlordiazepoxide), and barbiturates like Nembutal or mephobarbital (Mebaral)

- Anticonvulsant medications (drugs used to treat seizures) such as carbamazepine (Tegretol)

continued

- Antidepressant medications (drugs used to treat depression), including monoamine oxidase inhibitors (MAOI) like phenelzine(Nardil), which is especially dangerous with Demerol

- Tricyclic antidepressants like amitriptyline (Elavil)

- Muscle relaxants like Flexeril (cyclobenzaprine)

Naltrexone (Trexan, Revia): A narcotic antagonist and therefore can cancel the effects of these analgesics

Coumadin:

- Or other blood thinners, as the combination with narcotic may affect clotting times

Rifampin:

- An antibiotic used to treat bacterial infections

- Interacts with numerous medications, including analgesics, anticonvulsants, and antidepressants

Zidovudine:

- A drug used with other medications to treat HIV infection and can cause serious side effects in some patients when combined with aspirin, codeine, methadone, and morphine

Kava (*Piper methysticum*), chamomile (*Matricaria recutita*), lemon balm (*Melissa officinalis*):

- Or other herbal preparations that have calming or sedative effects, as they may intensify drowsiness and respiratory depression

Ginseng:

- An herbal stimulant; should also be avoided as it may interfere with the pain-relieving ability of narcotics

Combination Migraine Medications:

These are drugs that combine aspirin, acetaminophen, a narcotic analgesic, a sedative such as barbiturate, or an abortive like caffeine to provide better pain relief (see the "Combination Migraine Medications" sidebar).

A word of caution about caffeine: Caffeine is a vasoconstrictor, which means it may help to shrink dilated vessels. That is why it is added to the combination drugs and also why, when we have a cup of coffee or a glass of coke at the onset of a migraine attack, it might help to abort our attacks (see Chapter One for further information on the role of blood vessels in a migraine attack).

Combination Migraine Medications

Excedrin Migraine (aspirin, acetaminophen, and caffeine)

Fioricet (caffeine, a barbiturate, and acetaminophen)

Fiorinal (caffeine, a barbiturate, and aspirin)

Fiorinal with codeine (caffeine, a barbiturate, aspirin, and codeine)

Percocet (oxycodone and acetaminophen)

Percodan (oxycodone and aspirin)

Midrin: A combination of acetaminophen, isometheptene (causes narrowing of blood vessels), and dichloralphenazone (a sedative that depresses the CNS)

- Along with the preceding precautions for acetaminophen and CNS depressants, should not be taken if you have liver or kidney disease, circulation problems or coronary artery disease, hypertension, stomach or esophageal problems, or if you have had a heart attack or stroke.

Vicodin (hydrocodone and acetaminophen)

Vicoprofen (hydrocodone and ibuprofen)

As well, caffeine is a stimulant and besides giving us a spurt of energy, it increases peristalsis (the movement of food through our gut), which can help increase the absorption of our oral medications, and relieve symptoms of bloating, feelings of fullness, and nausea and vomiting.

The downside of caffeine is that it can cause rebound headaches (again, see Chapter Two for more information about rebound headaches). For this reason, many sources recommend that we keep our consumption of caffeine to a minimum.

Antiemetics

Once you and your doctor have settled on an analgesic, an antiemetic may be prescribed to treat the nausea and vomiting associated with your migraine attacks, be it mild or severe (see the "Common Antiemetics" sidebar). Some of these drugs may also contribute to your headache relief.

Common Antiemetics Used to Treat the Nausea and Vomiting Associated with Migraine Attacks

Dopamine antagonists: Are drugs that act in the brain to control nausea and vomiting such as:

- Phenothiazines, including Phenergan (Promethazine), Compazine (Prochlorperazine), and Thorazine (Chlorpromazine). Side effects of phenothiazines include hypotension, agitation, involuntary movements of the body, confusion, drowsiness, and fatigue.

- Tigan (Trimethobenzamide). Side effects include drowsiness, difficulty breathing, muscle spasms, seizures, and blurred vision.

- Reglan (metoclopramide). Is also a prokinetic drug, which means that it stimulates the muscles of the gastrointestinal tract and increases gastric emptying, which is often delayed during a migraine attack; besides nausea and vomiting, may relieve bloating (gastric distention) and a feeling of fullness that can be associated with a migraine attack. Side effects may include anxiety, rapid heart rate, muscle stiffness, or involuntary movements of your eyes (excessive blinking), jaw, mouth (lip smacking or mouth puckering), tongue (protruding), hands or feet (tapping or wiggling toes and fingers, flexing feet, and ankles). *A word of caution:* Tell your doctor immediately if you have any of these symptoms as they may be signs of a serious movement disorder known as Tardive Dyskinesia (risk increases the longer the drug is taken).

5-HT3 receptor antagonists: Are drugs that block serotonin receptors in the CNS and gastrointestinal tract, such as:

- Zofran (ondansetron). Side effects may include blurred vision, difficulty breathing, slow heart rate, shivering, anxiety, agitation, drowsiness, impaired thinking, and difficulty with urination.

At this point, it's important for you to note that except for Reglan, all of these antiemetics are available as rectal suppositories.

Abortive Drugs

If your migraine attacks are severe, and perhaps debilitating, in addition to an analgesic and an antiemetic, your doctor may prescribe a medication that can abort your headache at the onset. These medications can also help with associated symptoms like nausea and vomiting, and sensitivity to light. These medications include

Triptans: These drugs are serotonin receptor agonists, which means they copy the effects of serotonin and vasoconstrict blood vessels, as well as inhibit the release of inflammatory mediators that trigger much of the pain associated with your migraine attack (see Chapter One for more information on serotonin and inflammatory mediators).

- Because these medications cause vasoconstriction (and may cause spasm in the blood vessels), they should not be used if you have uncontrolled high blood pressure or diabetes, are at risk for stroke, or if you have heart disease.

- Side effects are less severe than those with ergot drugs (ergotamines) but can include tightness in the chest or throat, tingling in the fingers and toes, feeling of warmth, facial flushing, drowsiness, dizziness, weakness, and rapid heart rate.

- They aren't recommended for people with basilar or hemiplegic migraines (see Chapter Two for more information on types of migraines).

- Because triptans can increase serotonin levels in the brain and precipitate a condition known as *serotonin syndrome,* use them only with caution and under the direct supervision and control of your physician with any other drugs that increase serotonin levels, such as antidepressants like Prozac (fluoxetine) and Zoloft (sertaline).

- See the "Commonly Used Triptans" sidebar for commonly used triptans.

Commonly Used Triptans

Imitrex (sumatriptan): Longest triptan in use and is available as an oral tablet, nasal spray, rectal suppository, or subcutaneous (under the skin) injection.

Relpax (eletriptan): Only available as an oral tablet.

Maxalt (rizatriptan): Available as an oral tablet and a sublingual form.

Zomig (zolmitriptan): Available as an oral tablet, a sublingual form, and a nasal spray.

Axert (almotriptan): Only available as an oral tablet.

Amerge (naratriptan): Only available as an oral tablet, and although it takes longer to work, headaches are less likely to reoccur within twenty-four hours.

Frova (frovatriptan): Like Amerge, only available as an oral tablet, and although it takes longer to work, headaches are less likely to reoccur within twenty-four hours.

Treximet (combination of sumatriptan and the non-steroidal, anti-inflammatory drug, naproxen sodium): Some reports indicate that the combination of these two drugs in one pill may provide better relief for migraine pain than either drug alone. It is subject to the same side effects, complications, and precautions as all the other triptans and to the same side effects, complications, and precautions as all the other NSAIDs.

Zecuity: Recently approved by the FDA is a battery-operated skin patch indicated for acute treatment of migraine with or without aura in adults. Helps relieve headache pain and nausea. Subject to the same side effects, complications, and precautions as all the other triptans.

Ergotamines (ergots): These drugs constrict blood vessels and decrease blood flow to the brain and the body; therefore, they are not a good choice if you have uncontrollable high blood pressure and are at risk for a stroke or if you have heart, liver, or kidney disease; an irregular heartbeat (arrhythmia); an enlarged prostate; glaucoma; a recent infection; a bowel obstruction; or have had surgery.

- They should not be taken with other medications that decrease blood flow, including triptans, some antibiotics, some antidepressants, medications used to treat HIV or AIDS, and heart or blood pressure medications.

- They should not be taken if you are pregnant (can cause the baby to abort) or breast-feeding (can pass into breast milk).

- Side effects may include nausea and vomiting, dizziness, tingling sensations in the hands and feet, cold hands and feet, muscle cramps, and chest or abdominal pain.

- They were the first abortive drugs available (see the "Ergots That May Be Used" sidebar).

Ergots That May Be Used for Migraine Attacks

Dihydroergotamine (DHE): Available as an injection and as a nasal spray (Migranal).

Ergomar: Available as a sublingual form.

Ergotamine tartrate and caffeine (Cafergot, Migergot): Available as an oral tablet and a rectal suppository.

A word of caution: Excessive use of ergots can cause a dangerous decrease of blood supply to your extremities. It is important to tell your doctor immediately if you experience pain in your legs when walking, muscle pain, numbness, coldness, or abnormal paleness of your fingers or toes.

Prophylactic Drugs

If your migraine attacks occur more than two to three times a month, are severe and debilitating, and respond poorly to pain-relieving treatment, in addition to your other medications, your doctor may prescribe a preventative medication. These drugs are usually taken daily, and may take a month, or two, to reduce the frequency and severity of your migraine attacks. They include

Beta blockers: These drugs are commonly used to treat hypertension, angina, and irregular heart rhythms because they open up blood vessels and allow the heart to beat slower, with less force, and at a regular rate. It is thought that they help to prevent migraine attacks by stabilizing blood vessels and diminishing the effects that epinephrine and norepinephrine have on the nervous and vascular systems.

- Side effects may include dizziness, fatigue, exercise intolerance, insomnia, cold hands and feet, slow heart rate, shortness of breath, and impotence.

- Should not be used if you have asthma as can inhibit relaxation of bronchial muscle and exacerbate bronchospasm.

- Beta blockers used in the prevention of migraine attacks include Inderal (propanolol), Corgard (nadolol), Zebta (bisoprolol), Lopressor (metoprolol), and Blocadren (timolol).

Calcium channel blockers: These drugs are also used to treat high blood pressure and heart disease because they relax the cells in the blood vessel walls and prevent blood vessel spasm. Besides reducing blood vessel spasm, it is thought they help to prevent migraine attacks by decreasing inflammation in the brain cells.

- Side effects include fatigue, dizziness, fluid retention, and constipation.

- May not be the best choice if you have heart failure or a disturbance in the conduction system (electrical pathway) in the heart.

- Commonly used calcium channel blockers include verapamil (Calan, Isoptin).

Tricyclic antidepressants: These drugs alter the amount of serotonin and norepinephrine available for use in your body, and not only can affect your mood but also can reduce pain signals. They also can affect histamine release (histamine causes vasodilation), which can contribute to your pain.

- Side effects may include dry mouth, dry eyes, blurred vision, constipation, sexual dysfunction, drowsiness, increased appetite (weight gain), and an upset stomach.

- They can cause irregular heart rhythm, so they may not be best choice if you have heart disease.

Commonly used tricyclic antidepressants include Elavil (amitriptyline), Norpramin (desipramine), and Tofranil (imipramine). It's important to know that some other classes of antidepressants are thought to be less effective in migraine prevention, such as selective serotonin reuptake inhibitors (SSRIs) like Prozac (fluoxetine), which increase the amount of serotonin available for your body to use; serotonin and norepinephrine reuptake inhibitors (SNRIs) like Effexor (venlafaxine), which increase the amount of serotonin and norepinephrine available for your body to use; and norepinephrine-dopamine reuptake inhibitors like Bupropion (wellbutrin), which increase the amount of dopamine available for your body to use.

Anticonvulsants (anti-seizure drugs): The following two drugs affect the neurotransmitter gamma aminobutyric acid (GABA), which works to inhibit excessive brain activity and promote a state of calm:

- **Topamax (topiramate):** Side effects include drowsiness, fatigue, nausea and vomiting, weight loss, tingling in the arms and legs, poor memory, inability to concentrate, and less frequently, kidney stones.

- **Depakote (divalproex):** Side effects include nausea and vomiting, drowsiness, dizziness, hair loss, weight gain, and possible liver damage. Should not be taken if you have liver disease (regular liver function tests are recommended if you take this medication). Known to cause birth defects, so you should not take this drug if you're pregnant, or thinking of becoming pregnant.

Methysergide: This is an ergot alkaloid (related to the ergotamines discussed in abortive medications). Thought to vasoconstrict (narrow) blood vessels in the head and reduce the throbbing pain associated with vascular headaches like migraine.

- Because of numerous serious side effects (too many to mention here), it is taken only under a doctor's close supervision to help prevent migraine headaches when other drugs such as beta blockers fail to work.

Botox (botulinum toxin type A): Is a bacterial protein—recently approved by the FDA for chronic migraine that occurs fifteen or more days per month and lasts longer than four hours each day—that is thought to relax muscles and suppress the transmission of nerve impulses, or pain messages, sent to the brain. Reviews are mixed, but some studies show that Botox can reduce the number of headache days per month for chronic migraineurs.

- Injections are administered to affected muscles in your forehead, scalp, temple, and neck. Injections may take two to three months to work, may have to be repeated every two to three months to be effective, and should be administered by a doctor trained in Botox treatment for migraine disease.

- Side effects may include pain in the injected area for a few days, sagging eyelids, excessive muscle weakness, muscle spasm, difficulty breathing, talking or swallowing, chest pain, and irregular heartbeat.

What Else You Need to Know About Your Medication

As you can see, there are numerous side effects and contraindications associated with the drugs we ingest to stop or prevent our migraine attacks. For this reason, you need to communicate with your doctor on a regular basis about your progress. For example:

- Has the medication you're taking made you feel better, or worse?

- If you're taking a preventative medication, are your migraine attacks occurring more or less often?

The first goal of any drug therapy is to provide maximum relief for any discomfort, at the smallest dose possible, and with the fewest number of side effects. This is known as the *therapeutic dose*.

For example: I remember when a cardiologist tried to switch me from Calan (which I was taking at the time to control palpitations and a rapid heart rate associated with my mitral valve prolapse) to Inderal. He thought, and rightly so, that the beta blocker would be better at preventing my migraine attacks because it would lessen the effects that epinephrine and other stress hormones had on my body. After only two low doses of Inderal, though, I was so dizzy that I could not stand up, let alone function in any capacity. Obviously, that drug was not for me.

The second goal of drug therapy should be to wean off unnecessary or more dangerous medications (those with harmful side effects) once your migraine attacks have improved. This is the point where you and your doctor need to work together to reduce the amount of medication you require. You should never discontinue any of your prescribed medications without your doctor's knowledge.

Latest Research and Potential New Drugs and Treatments You Might Want to Know About

It seems every time you turn on the television or look at the Internet, supposed state of the art treatments for migraine headaches pop up. Beware. At this point, there are no miracle cures for our disease.

However, as research continues, more and more drugs are being tested with the hope of introducing them on to the market. Some of these drugs include Tezampanel (NGX424), which affects the role of the neurotransmitter; glutamate; those that target the inflammatory mediator known as substance P; and more recently, drugs that address the connection between migraine disease and the digestive system (the gut-brain connection). In addition, as research continues on the genetic component of migraines, it is thought that a new generation of drugs may be able to affect a gene called TRESK, which is believed to be fundamental in causing migraines (see Chapter One for more information on neurotransmitters and substance P, and see Chapter Two for more information on TRESK).

Looking Back and Glimpsing Ahead

In this chapter, you read about numerous medications available to treat our disease, including analgesics, antiemetics, abortive, and preventative drugs. Now that you are aware of the action, side effects, and contraindications of the drugs you take, let's apply this information to your wellness plan.

First, to avoid rebound headaches, do not exceed the recommended dose or take the medication more often than your doctor or the label on the container recommends. If a medication is not working for you, ask your doctor to switch you to one that might be more effective.

Second, if the route of administration is not working for you, ask your doctor to switch you to another one. For example, if you cannot keep down the pills you swallow, a nasal spray or suppository would be more beneficial.

Lastly, if the frequency and severity of your migraine attacks persist no matter what, or how much medication you ingest, you may want to do what I did when I found I couldn't keep running on adrenalin and popping Imitrex to maintain the hectic lifestyle I loved. Even though at that time, I did not believe in the benefits of acupuncture or other integrative therapies that evolved from Eastern medicine, I gave them a try. I am forever grateful that I did.

In the chapters ahead, as I mention in Chapter Three, I talk about a number of treatments and therapies like acupuncture, meditation, mind-body exercises, and energy-healing techniques that can help you relax, stabilize your serotonin levels, increase your endorphins, and decrease the frequency and severity of your migraine attacks. As well, I show you how integration of these modalities into your wellness plan can enhance the effect of the medication you take, and reduce the amount you require.

PART TWO

Traditional Chinese Medicine and Migraine Disease

CHAPTER FIVE

Traditional Chinese Medicine (TCM)

WHEN I FIRST MET Dr. Mao, my knowledge of Traditional Chinese Medicine (TCM) was limited. I was skeptical about making an appointment and apprehensive about keeping it. However, my husband gave me no choice. He was determined to do whatever it took to get me off the amount of medication I consumed, and what didn't seem to be doing a darn thing to help get rid of my migraine attacks, or relieve my agony. If that meant driving from the desert to Santa Monica on his only day off for weeks at a time, to him it was worth the chore.

As I sat in Dr. Mao's office and waited for his entrance, I wanted to bolt. My temples had started to throb, and all I could think about were the needles that were about to be poked into my pain. Amazing though, once he walked in, a sense of calmness began to wash over me. Suddenly, I was aware of the soft colors in the room, the soothing music in the background; and when he spoke in a gentle voice, my breathing stilled, and my heart rate slowed.

For at least an hour, he spoke with my husband and me and asked many of the questions I will share with you in Chapter

Seven. When he finished, he escorted me to a small room with the same soft colors and soothing music in the background. I sat on a narrow bed, more like a comfortable massage table, and he proceeded with my physical exam. Holding both my hands at the wrist where he could feel my pulses, he looked into my eyes and asked me to stick out my tongue. That was it. In less than ten minutes, the exam was over.

Now it was time for acupuncture. I didn't have to undress—just took off my flip-flops and pulled up my tee-shirt to expose my belly. Somewhat nervous, I laid down on the bed with a pillow under my head and one beneath my knees. I recall that I flinched at the first needle, but that was because I was scared it might hurt. After that, I felt nothing but a nice warm feeling, enhanced by one heat lamp over my feet and one over my belly. He vacated the room, and I fell asleep. An hour later, I woke to the sound of my snores and a wonderful feeling of contentment. My headache had disappeared, and for those few moments, nothing could disturb the peace of my soul.

Over the years, as the benefits of my treatments increased, my curiosity about TCM grew. As ingrained in Western medicine as I was, I wanted to know at least something about Eastern medicine and how it worked.

I did some research, and the results were enlightening. In the next few chapters, I will share with you what I learned. The information I discuss is not meant to be an in-depth study of TCM, but rather a simple explanation of the guiding principles that, whether or not you see a doctor of TCM, can be applied to your path to wellness. For a more detailed discussion on any of the aspects involved, please refer to *Secrets of Self-Healing* (Avery, 2008) by Dr. Mao, along with the "References" section at the end of this book.

I discovered that TCM is a naturalistic philosophy of health and medicine that looks at the interrelationship of our body, mind, and spirit. Every human being is considered unique.

The patient and the doctor work together to maintain and sustain good health. The focus of the relationship is on the prevention of disease and the concept of wellness (if you're fortunate, as I have been, you may find a doctor of conventional Western medicine or Holistic Medicine who also advocates prevention and wellness).

Disease is viewed as a life out of balance, and people are encouraged to take care of themselves before a problem arises. This requires individuals to take responsibility for their own health and to maintain a healthy lifestyle that includes exercise, diet, and practices such as meditation to reduce the effects of stress and to balance the energy centers in their bodies.

What Is Chi?

Chi is considered to be the vital energy force that flows through our organs and muscles and permeates every tissue and cell in our body. It is thought to be responsible for all the workings of our mind and body, including respiration (breathing), circulation of blood and fluids through our body, digestion and absorption of the food we eat, and elimination of our waste products. Chi also allows our five senses (hearing, sight, smell, taste, and touch) to perform their functions.

Chi is referred to as the breath of life in all living organisms. The absence of chi is death. Chi, or the energy in our body, may appear in various forms. These forms depend on internal factors in our body such as our physical, emotional, and spiritual state, and external factors such as the climate and our environment. Some examples of these forms are the heat associated with fever, liquid forms like diarrhea or a runny nose when circulation of fluid is affected, and sweaty palms during times of stress.

Chi flows through our body via canals called *channels*, or *meridians*. When I discuss acupuncture in Chapter Eight, I will talk more about these channels. For now, all you need to know is that there are twelve main channels and each corresponds to a particular organ network system (see discussion on the Organ Network System later in this chapter). Blockage or imbalance of the flow of energy in these channels, as described by Dr. Mao in *Secrets of Self-Healing* (Avery, 2008), may result in a number of symptoms (see Table 5.1).

What Is Yin, and What Is Yang?

Yin and yang are opposite, although complementary, energies essential to all facets of life. In an effort to maintain equilibrium, the energy is dynamic, or constantly changing, rather than static. For example, take our human body. If we get too hot and develop a fever, we sweat and cool down. If we're too cold, we shiver and generate heat.

Besides cold and hot, yin/yang is the way of things such as earth and heaven, moon and sun, dark and light, night and day, slow and fast, negative and positive, water and fire, interior and exterior, feminine and masculine, autumn/winter and spring/summer, sadness and happiness, and love and hate. Where there is an up, there is a down; a back cannot exist without a front. We cannot know joy if we have not experienced sorrow. And so it goes, on and on.

The important thing here is that, in health and disease, when our yin and yang are in balance and harmony, we will enjoy good health and a sense of peace. When our yin and yang are out of balance, our health will be affected.

TABLE 5.1: SYMPTOMS THAT MAY BE RELATED TO THE BLOCKAGE OR IMBALANCE OF ENERGY FLOW IN THE TWELVE CHANNELS

CHANNEL	SYMPTOMS RELATED TO BLOCKAGE OF ENERGY FLOW
Lung	Sore throat, congestion, cough, coughing up blood, a feeling of fullness in your chest, and pain in your clavicle (collar bone), shoulder, back, and inside of your arms
Large Intestine	Watery nasal discharge, nosebleed, toothaches, sore and congested throat, pain in the neck or front part of your upper arms or shoulders, noisy or rumbling intestines, abdominal pain, constipation, diarrhea or dysentery
Stomach	Noisy or growly intestines, abdominal distention or bloating, vomiting, increased appetite, nosebleed, Bell's palsy, fever, sore and congested throat, mental disturbance, and pain in your chest, stomach, abdomen, or outer part of your leg
Spleen	Burping (belching), bloating (abdominal distention), vomiting, stomach pain, jaundice, loose stools, sluggishness, general malaise, stiffness and pain at the back of your tongue, swelling and coldness in your inner thighs and knees
Heart	Palpitations, chest pain, rib pain, pain in the insides of your upper arms, dry throat, thirst, insomnia, night sweats, feverishness in your palms
Small Intestine	Yellow (jaundice) in the whites of your eyes, deafness, swelling of your cheeks, sore throat, distention and pain in your lower abdomen, frequent urination, pain along the back and outer parts of your shoulders and arms
Bladder	Yellow (jaundice) in the whites of your eyes, deafness, swelling of your cheeks, sore throat, distention and pain in your lower abdomen, frequent urination, pain along the back and outer parts of your shoulders and arms

continued

continued

TABLE 5.1: SYMPTOMS THAT MAY BE RELATED TO THE BLOCKAGE OR IMBALANCE OF ENERGY FLOW IN THE TWELVE CHANNELS	
CHANNEL	**SYMPTOMS RELATED TO BLOCKAGE OF ENERGY FLOW**
Kidney	Frequent urination, bedwetting, nocturnal emissions, impotence, irregular menstruation, dry tongue, congested and swelling and sore throat, asthma, swelling, low-back pain, pain along your spinal column and inner thighs, weakness of the legs, feverish sensation in the soles of your feet
Pericardium	Chest pain, stifling feeling in your chest, palpitations, mental restlessness, mental disturbance, flushed face, swelling under your arm, spasm of your arms, feverishness in your palms
Triple Warmer	Abdominal distention, bed wetting, difficulty with urination, deafness, ear ringing, swelling of your cheeks, congested and sore throat; pain in the outer corners of your eyes, backs of your ears, shoulders, and outer parts of your arms and elbows
Gall Bladder	Headache, blurred vision, bitter taste in your mouth, swelling and pain in your collarbone; pain in the outer corners of your eyes, jaw, armpits (axillae), the outer part of your chest, ribs, thighs, and calves
Liver	Headache on top of your scalp (crown of your head), dry throat, hiccups, fullness in your chest, hernia, pain in your low back and lower abdomen, bedwetting, difficulty urinating, mental disturbances

Where yin and yang describe the process of energy evolution and polarization, the five phases of energy represent the way in which our chi energy is transformed to maintain a balance between our internal and external environments (*homeostasis*). Each of us is believed to be a customized blend of the influences of these five phases.

The five phases are wood, fire, earth, metal, and water. The flow of energy is cyclical, according to the four seasons, and interactive. Besides a specific season, each of these phases is associated with an organ network system (ONS), and other things such as color, emotion, taste, smell, body opening and sense organ, excreted fluid, climate, and outward manifestation (see Table 5.2). As well, like yin and yang, each phase has both dynamic and static characteristics.

The Wood Phase

The wood phase (refer to Table 5.2) is associated with the wind of spring and involves the aspects of youth, sexuality, growth, and harmony. The energy flow is strong-rooted, rising, exhilarating, and expansive (spring fever). It gives us the urge to procreate, move our muscles, activate tissues, set goals, and make decisions. The wood phase corresponds to our liver-gall bladder network and controls many of our body's basic functions, as well as the smooth flow of chi.

The Fire Phase

The fire phase (Table 5.2) is associated with the heat of summer and maximum growth. The energy flow is upward, hot, explosive, and excitable. Connected to love, compassion, and generosity, it gives us the ability to socialize and form warm, human relationships.

The fire phase corresponds with our heart, small intestine, pericardium, and triple warmer and controls aspects of digestion, as well as the circulation of fluids. Because the mind and spirit reside in the heart, fire also controls our memory, thinking, and dreaming.

The Earth Phase

The earth phase (Table 5.2) is associated with the dampness of late summer, or harvest time. The energy flow is downward and is balancing and anchoring. It gives us a feeling of completeness and the ability to be grounded, centered, nurturing, and compassionate (hence the phrase "mother earth"). The earth phase corresponds with our spleen, pancreas, and stomach and controls the breakdown of the foods we eat.

The Metal Phase

The metal phase (Table 5.2) is associated with the dryness of autumn, and the aspects of conduction, contraction, consolidation, organization, and change. The energy flow is inward for accumulation and storage. It gives us the ability to be well balanced, organized, self-disciplined, and conscientious. The metal phase corresponds with our lungs and large intestine and controls respiration, perspiration, and the removal of waste from our body.

The Water Phase

The water phase (Table 5.2) is associated with the cold of winter and the aspects of quiet, silence, waiting, rest, flexibility, and great power. The energy flow is downward, enduring, and cooling. It gives us the ability to be fearless, determined, and to persevere through hardships to achieve our goals. The water phase corresponds with our kidneys and bladder and controls fluid metabolism, as well as the regulation of the endocrine system through our adrenal glands.

The Relationship Between the Five Phases and Disease

Each of the five phases acts upon one another to keep the system in balance. For example, wood feeds fire, fire generates ashes and

TABLE 5.2: THE FIVE ELEMENTS AND THEIR RELATIONSHIP TO THE ORGAN NETWORK SYSTEMS, ALONG WITH THEIR ASSOCIATED QUALITIES

QUALITY	Wood	Fire	Earth	Metal	Water
SEASON	Spring	Summer	Late summer or harvest	Autumn	Winter
ONS	Liver–Gall Bladder	Heart–Small Intestine–Pericardium–Triple Warmer	Spleen–Pancreas–Stomach	Lungs–Large Intestine	Kidney–Bladder
COLOR	Green	Red	Yellow	White	Black
EMOTION	Anger	Joy	Worry	Grief	Fear
TASTE	Sour	Bitter	Sweat	Pungent or spicy	Salty
SMELL	Rancid	Scorched	Fragrant	Putrid	Rotten
BODY OPENING	Eyes	Throat	Mouth	Nose	Ears, urethra, anus
FLUID SECRETED	Tears	Sweat	Saliva	Mucous	Urine
CLIMATE	Wind	Hot	Damp	Dry	Cold
MANIFESTATION	Nails and sight	Tongue and pulse	Lips	Skin and body hair	Hair of head

forms earth, metal is heated inside the earth and produces water vapor, water nourishes wood, and the process is repeated. This generating cycle is known as the *shen cycle.*

The *ko,* or controlling, cycle demonstrates how the elements restrict one another. Wood can penetrate earth's soil. Earth can obstruct the flow of water. Water is able to douse fire. Fire melts metal, and metal cuts wood.

It's important for you to understand that an individual's good health is dependent on the harmonious balance of the influences of all the five phases, which shift from one to another, in response to various stimuli throughout the day. If one of our emotions becomes dominant—for example, anger, which is a manifestation of the wood phase—the cycle of the five phase system is disrupted. Our internal energies stagnate and disease occurs.

The Organ Network System

Another important aspect is that in TCM, the definition of an organ is not limited to the physical organ within our body. Rather, our organs are seen as an entire network of energy systems, which are responsible for everything that occurs in our body, including the physical, emotional, and spiritual qualities we possess. When imbalance between our organ network systems and the external environment exists, sickness and disease appears.

The Liver-Gallbladder Network

In TCM, the primary functions of the liver are to regulate the smooth flow of energy (chi) and blood throughout the body. The liver also stores and filters blood (removes bacteria and maintains the body's defense systems); produces bile and aids in the breakdown, absorption, and storage of fats; synthesizes proteins including those responsible for holding fluid in the vascular spaces and the clotting of blood; converts glucose to glycogen for energy; and aids in the detoxification of hormones and drugs, while regulating some functions of the nervous system like muscular movement and tension. The gall bladder is responsible for the storage and secretion of bile and the participation in digestion. It also works with the lymphatic system to clear toxic byproducts of metabolism.

As mentioned in Table 5.2, wood is the phase associated with the liver-gall bladder network and anger is the emotion. When we become angry, energy is directed upward to our head and shoulders. We may lash out with the explosiveness of the wind in the spring; hence the verbal expression tied to the phase is shouting.

If the energy of our liver-gall bladder network is depleted, we may be overcome by indecisiveness, fatigue, and fear. We may appear to be without direction in our life and unable to express anger. If our energy is congested or stagnant, we may be arrogant, over-controlling, and have an angry disposition. As well, we may be workaholics or have addictive personalities.

Diseases, or imbalances, associated with the liver-gall bladder network may reflect the following symptoms: migraine or tension headaches; hypertension; eye disorders such as blurred vision and glaucoma; dizziness; redness of the face and eyes; yellow eyes (jaundice); sinus problems; menstrual difficulties, including cysts or fibroids, painful periods, and heavy bleeding; outbursts of anger, impatience, frustration, inability to relax, irritation; belching, bloating, nausea; and soft-ridged nails.

The Heart-Small Intestine Network

The heart is considered to be the control center of our body. That is because it controls the circulation of our blood and the regulation of our blood vessels, and it is the home of our spirit, or divine energy. When our energy descends downward to our other organs, it functions as our balancing center. When it ascends upward to our brain, it functions as our mind. The small intestine separates pure nutrient energy from the impure, and transports it downward.

As mentioned in Table 5.2, fire is the phase associated with the heart-small intestine network and joy is the emotion. Too much joy causes our energy to disperse. We may be left exhausted as in the hot days of summer, or giddy and weak; hence the vocal expression associated with this phase is laughter.

If the energy of our heart-small intestine is depleted, we may suffer from anxiety, restlessness, insomnia, and excessive dreaming. We may be easily excitable and stimulated and have a nervous laugh. Or we may be emotionally cold and devoid of feelings. Because speech corresponds to the heart and mind, we may talk too much and too fast, or stutter.

Diseases or imbalances associated with our heart-small intestine network may reflect the following symptoms: palpitations, dizziness and fainting, hypertension, heart problems, varicose and spider veins, sores on the mouth and tongue, constipation, diarrhea, abdominal pain, blood in the urine, and painful urination. And because the heart is the control center of the body, any disease affecting it will also disturb all other functions.

The Pericardium-Triple Warmer Network

The pericardium is the fatty membrane, which protects our heart. As well, it maintains the order of our heart's energy by protecting it from damage by excessive emotional energies generated by the other organ systems.

The triple warmer consists of the upper warmer, which involves our heart and lungs; the middle warmer, which involves our stomach, spleen, and liver; and the lower warmer, which involves our kidneys, large and small intestines, and bladder. The energy network of the triple warmer extends through our body cavities and, combined with the fatty deposits, protects our organs and regulates our body temperature. It also works with the respective organ systems to govern our respiration, control our digestion and distribution of nutrients, eliminate our waste, and regulate our sexual and reproductive functions.

Like the heart-small intestine network, fire is the phase associated with our pericardium triple-warmer network (see Table 5.2). All the corresponding characteristics—for example, the emotion joy—are the same.

Diseases or imbalances of our pericardium-triple network may reflect the following symptoms: fever, chills, extremes of hot and cold, dizziness, loss of voice, and burning with urination.

The Spleen-Pancreas-Stomach Network

In TCM, the spleen is given the same functions that Western medicine gives the pancreas. The primary function of our spleen is considered to be the transformation, distribution, and storage of nutrients and energy for our entire body. The spleen works with the stomach to perform the functions of digestion and absorption of the nutrients we ingest. As well, the spleen regulates our blood volume and has an essential role in our imagination and creativity.

The stomach governs digestion. Where the spleen is in charge of distributing and circulating the nutrients from food, the stomach is the depository of nourishment for our body. Therefore, any disease in the stomach will be reflected in the other organs in the network.

As mentioned in Table 5.2, earth is the phase associated with the spleen-pancreas-stomach network and worry is the emotion.

Excessive worry causes our energy to slow down or stagnate. We may be left lazy and inactive, unable to do the smallest of tasks as in the damp, or humid, days of late summer. The vocal expression associated with this phase is singing.

If the energy of our spleen-pancreas-stomach network is depleted, we may suffer from pensiveness, cloudy thinking, and may overindulge in studying or other intellectual endeavors. We may gain weight easily and lose it with difficulty. As well, our bodies have a tendency to make excessive mucous.

Diseases or imbalances of the spleen-pancreas-stomach network may reflect the following symptoms: indigestion, abdominal pain, gas and bloating, acid reflux, lack of appetite, diarrhea, constipation, insomnia, fatigue, and an excessive collection of mucous in the lungs or sinuses.

The Lung-Large Intestine Network

The primary function of our lung is to control breathing and gas exchange with the external environment (respiration). The lung also plays a crucial role in our immunity, as it is the first line of defense against the invasion of foreign particles and pathogens in inspired air and in our blood.

The large intestine is responsible for the final absorption of water and nutrients, and the storage and removal of waste from our body. As well, it works with our lung to maintain a healthy immune system.

As mentioned in Table 5.2, metal is the phase associated with our lung-large intestine network and sadness is the emotion. Grief causes our energy to stop. We may feel cut off from life, like the leaves that fall in autumn. Tears wash away our pain and sorrow; hence the vocal expression tied to this phase is weeping.

If the energy of our lung-large intestine is depleted, we may be overly critical and have a problem letting go. Persistent sadness may leave us exhausted and wear down our body's immune system.

Diseases or imbalances of our lung-large intestine network may reflect the following symptoms: shortness of breath, cough, asthma, sinus problems, skin breakouts, allergies, food sensitivities, colitis, upper-back pain, and constipation.

The Kidney-Bladder Network

In TCM, the function of the kidney is two-fold. First, it controls the amount of fluid in our body. Some fluid is released with respiration and perspiration (sweat) and evacuated with stool, but most of the fluid descends downward from the kidney to our bladder for storage and release.

Second, our kidney stores two kinds of essence. One is the basic nourishment of life, which is derived from food and air, and can be released as necessary to any organ in the network. And second is reproductive essence, which is the basic substance of our human reproduction.

As mentioned in Table 5.2, water is the phase associated with our kidney-bladder network and fear is the emotion. When fear predominates, our energy sinks. We may be immobilized or feel frozen, as in the frigid days of winter. The vocal expression associated with this phase is groaning.

If the energy of our kidney-bladder network is depleted, we may be anxious, withdrawn, and fearful. As well, we may be subject to paranoia.

Disease or imbalances of our kidney-bladder network may reflect the following symptoms: edema (water retention), urinary problems such as frequency and retention, painful joints, brittle bones, sexual disorders, irregular menstruation, impaired hearing, ringing in the ears, dark circles or pouches under the eyes, and forgetfulness.

Looking Back and Glimpsing Ahead

In this chapter, you learned that TCM is a naturalistic philosophy of health and medicine that looks at the interrelationship of a person's body, mind, and spirit. In the process, you learned about the nature of energy. You discovered that if our energy is balanced and in harmony with our external environment, we have good health. When an imbalance of energy occurs, we're subject to disease.

Now that you understand the relationship of energy to health and disease, we can apply the knowledge you have gained in the chapters ahead.

CHAPTER SIX

Causes of Disharmony and Disease

IN CHAPTER FIVE, YOU discovered that in TCM, good health is dependent upon the smooth flow of chi, the balance of yin and yang, the influences of the five phases, and the balance between our organ network systems and our external environment. However, you need to know a few more things.

As Dr. Mao explains in the *Secrets of Self-Healing* (Avery, 2008), while TCM recognizes the role of germs and bacteria, as well as other factors like heredity (genetics), parasites (animal and insect borne), traumatic injuries, faulty diets, destructive lifestyles, mechanical or radiation damage, and epidemics, as causes of disorders in the human body, it is believed that certain conditions are necessary for disease and disharmony to occur. First, there must be a receptive host, which is a body out of balance. Second, because the weakened body is unable to protect itself, it cannot adjust to external and internal influences (referred to as *pathogens*) and therefore allows them to cause damage.

The External Influences, or Causes, of Disease

The external causes of disease are related to the seasonal weather or climatic changes, which correspond with the five phases I talk about in Chapter Five (refer to Table 5.2). They are wind, heat, dampness, dryness, and cold. Although each of these conditions can affect our body during any of the seasons, disease is more likely to occur during the related season, unseasonably related weather, or from artificially created environments such as air conditioning, central heating, microwave radiation, fluorescent lights, smoking, and polluted air or water.

Wind

Spring, a time of sudden growth and rapid change, is the season associated with the unpredictable, rising and falling gusts of wind. During the months of spring, the breeze can also be calm, mild, and pleasant. When wind occurs in another season, it takes on the energies of that season—for example, the hot wind of summer, the damp wind of late summer, the dry wind of autumn, and the cold wind of winter.

When wind finds its way into our body, it causes disorders such as flu and the common cold. Like the wind, our symptoms tend to wander and change or suddenly disappear. Characteristics of a wind attack include headache, body aches, fever and chills, stuffy nose, sinus congestion, and cough.

As well, you need to be aware that a wind environment is created inside our body when too much wind energy accumulates in an internal organ system. The excess of wind energy may cause serious imbalances in the vital energy of that system. The imbalance may move suddenly to another organ system and may overstimulate or suppress it. Excess liver wind causes energy to rise to our head and stimulates symptoms like headache, dizziness, insomnia, and blurred vision.

Heat

Summer, a season full of hot air temperatures that may prevail over a long period of time, is associated with sweltering heat. Although heat is specific to summer, it may combine with the dryness of autumn, or environmental energies such as central heating to cause a form of dry heat. *Fire,* an extreme form of heat, can be brought on by an excessive imbalance of energy related to any of the seasonal energies—for example, the dampness or humidity connected to late summer.

The nature of heat is to rise and move outward toward the surface. It may be discharged as sweat, or seen as a red face and eyes, skin ulcers, redness on the tip of our tongue, a full and bounding pulse, or signs of inflammation like redness, heat, pain, and swelling in an affected area.

When heat attacks our body, it increases our metabolism and dilates our vessels. Characteristics of an attack include fever, irritability, decreased appetite, nausea, vomiting, diarrhea, headache, thirst, profuse sweating, and in severe cases associated with sunstroke, delirium, dizziness, and unconsciousness. When combined with dampness or humidity, additional symptoms may include a heavy feeling in our head and whole body, stuffiness and a feeling of fullness in our chest, and abdominal distention (bloating).

As well, you need to be aware that a heat environment can be created inside our body with exercise, the ingestion of warm or spicy foods, alcoholic beverages, and drugs such as amphetamines. If an imbalanced body already has excessive heat, these factors may exacerbate these disorders and symptoms.

Dampness

Late summer, a season where rain, morning mist, and damp ground may prevail, is associated with humidity and the stagnant, heavy, air. Dampness is often combined with cold, heat, or wind.

When dampness seeps into our body, stagnation and sluggishness of our circulation occurs. The movement tends to be downward and gives us a feeling of fullness and heaviness in our abdomen and lower extremities. Other characteristics may include fatigue, lethargy, shortness of breath, rheumatic pains, stiff and swollen joints, and bloating.

As well, you need to be aware that a damp environment may be created inside our body with the ingestion of starchy foods, watery fruits and vegetables, and dairy products. In addition, drugs such as steroids and birth control pills can aggravate our symptoms.

Dryness

Autumn, a season where insufficient moisture in the air may prevail, is associated with dryness. When dryness occurs in another season, it takes on the energies of that season—for example, dry heat, dry cold, and dry wind.

The tendency of dryness is to consume our body fluids. Dehydration prevails and is evidenced by chapped lips, brittle hair and nails, dry and cracked skin, dry eyes and nostrils, dry mouth, and decreased sweat and urine production. Our lungs are particularly susceptible to dryness. Since they are paired with the large intestine, besides respiratory disorders, we may experience hard stools and constipation.

As well, you need to be aware that a dry environment can be created inside our body with the ingestion of hot and spicy foods and drugs such as nicotine, diuretics, and antihistamines. Because these substances can generate heat or deplete moisture, they will worsen our disorders and magnify our symptoms.

Cold

Winter, a season where low air temperatures may prevail over a long period of time, is associated with cold. Although cold is prevalent in winter, it may occur in other seasons like the cold, dryness of autumn or combine with environmental energies such as air conditioning.

When cold penetrates our body, it decreases our metabolism and causes our blood vessels to narrow. Symptoms such as paleness, chills, abdominal and joint pain, back pain, fatigue, frequent and clear urination, gas, loose stools, and loss of sexual vitality may occur.

As well, you need to be aware that a cold environment can be created inside our body by the ingestion of raw foods, refrigerated or ice-cold beverages, and ice cream. Drugs such as aspirin, antibiotics, and antacids have a cold influence and may affect our digestion.

At this point, it is interesting to note that in conventional Western medicine many of these external influences are believed to trigger our migraine attacks or cause physical, chemical, or environmental stress. As I talk about in Chapter Three, stress affects our sympathetic nervous system, makes us more susceptible to our triggers, and can intensify our migraine attacks. As well, chronic stress can deplete our stress hormones, sex hormones, and levels of neurotransmitters like serotonin and make us more prone to migraine attacks.

The Internal Influences, or Causes, of Disease

The internal causes of disease are believed to be associated with emotional damage. It is thought that once an emotion damages a respective organ network system, it causes imbalance and disorder in other organ network systems. The resultant emotional stress can cause stagnation of energy flow and lead to physical breakdown.

The emotions involved are anger, joy, worry, grief, and fear. Like the external influences previously addressed, they are related to the five phases I talk about in Chapter Five (refer to Table 5.2).

Anger

Anger causes liver chi to rise to our shoulders, neck, and head. The rush of energy can give us confidence and the ability to exert authority. However, when our anger is inappropriate, excessive, and prolonged, it causes a flare up of liver fire, which, in turn, may cause heart fire.

Anger embraces several other related emotions such as rage, fury, irritability, frustration, resentment, and bitterness. Damaging effects of these emotions include headache, dizziness, high blood pressure, tension and pain in our neck and shoulders, and in extreme cases, stroke and heart attack.

Joy

Joy affects our heart. When one is at peace and filled with happiness, chi is calm and opens our heart to promote acceptance and love. When excessive joy or excitement prevails, our metabolic rate speeds up. Heart energy is dispersed and affects our other network systems as well.

Damaging effects of too much joy include palpitations, dizziness, and fatigue. Other manifestations include excessive giggling, talkativeness, and giddiness. Some studies have shown that people who talk too fast have an increased incidence of heart disease and stroke.

Shock (Fright)

Shock weakens the chi of our heart-small intestine network. The unexpected nature of the fright, or shock to our system, scatters energy and injures our heart and kidneys. Often diseases or disorders experienced by an individual can be traced back to the time of the shock.

Worry (Rumination, Pensiveness)

Worry knots or congeals energy and affects our spleen-pancreas-stomach network. If our spleen-pancreas-stomach network cannot perform normal functions, digestive problems such as ulcers and indigestion occur.

Extreme worry, or pensiveness, can trap energy within our brain and lead to excessive thinking, brooding, insomnia, and apathy. It can also affect our lung and lead to anxiety, breathlessness, and problems in the neck and shoulders.

Grief

Grief, or sadness, the heaviest of all emotional energies, affects our lung-large intestine network. When sadness promotes caring and compassion, it can be a healthy emotion. However, when it is excessive, or chronic, it dissolves chi and consumes our energy.

Damaging effects from too much sadness include depression, tiredness, breathlessness, and respiratory disorders such as colds and bronchitis. As well, extreme grief can impair our resistance to more serious illnesses like cancer.

Fear

Fear causes chi to descend and affects our kidneys. A healthy dose of fear can be a great motivator—for example, the instinct necessary for survival. However, an excess of fear, such as a fear of failure, can be inhibitory and keep us from pursuing a desired career or other goals.

Damaging effects of fear may include bedwetting (in children), involuntary bowel movements and urinary incontinence in adults during extreme fright, anxiety, and pain or weakness in the lower back and legs. Chronic fear may lead to renal failure and permanent kidney damage.

At this point, it is interesting to note that in conventional Western medicine many of these internal influences are thought to cause emotional stress. Apart from the effects of stress I just mentioned and talked about in Chapter Three, chronic emotional stress can influence the immune system. For example, laughter and joy have a positive effect on immunity. Grief and sorrow weaken immunity.

Looking Back and Glimpsing Ahead

In this chapter, you learned that in TCM, for disease and disharmony to occur, there has to be a body out of balance. The weakened body cannot defend itself and, therefore, allows external and internal influences to damage organ systems and cause disease.

You also learned that in conventional Western medicine, many of these external and internal influences are considered to be triggers for our migraine attacks or can cause physical, chemical, environmental, or emotional stress.

Now, let's apply this information to our wellness plans. In TCM, a person is encouraged to incorporate treatments and therapies like acupuncture, meditation, and mind-body exercises into their lifestyle to keep their energy centers balanced and prevent disease.

In Chapters Eight and Nine, I show you how we can integrate these same therapies into our wellness plans to keep our sympathetic nervous system balanced and reduce the physiological response of our bodies to stress, stabilize our serotonin levels, and prevent a number of our migraine attacks.

CHAPTER SEVEN

The TCM View of Migraine Disease

It is important for you to know that although TCM recognizes genetics, vascular irregularities, neurotransmitters, and inflammatory mediators as contributing factors to the devastating headache associated with migraine disease, it does not focus on these etiological origins. Rather, TCM looks at migraine disease, as it does every other disease, as a disorder of the body as a whole.

As you discovered in Chapters Five and Six, if a body is balanced and in harmony with nature and its surroundings, it is strong enough to defend itself against external and internal influences. When imbalance or disharmony occurs, these external and internal influences become pathogens, attack organ network systems, and cause disease.

In TCM, the headache associated with migraine disease is believed to be related to an imbalance in one or more of the following organ-network systems.

Liver-Gall Bladder Organ Network System

The liver-gall bladder is the primary organ network system believed to be responsible for our migraine headaches. An imbalance in yin/yang energy is thought to cause a disruption in the flow of chi, blood stasis, and the accumulation of heat:

- When external influences like wind-cold, wind-heat, wind-damp or internal influences such as anger, frustration, and impatience disrupt the ability of our liver to move chi smoothly, chi and blood can become blocked and stagnate.

- Stagnation can cause heat, or an excess of liver energy, to accumulate. Heat rises to our head and manifests as pain. (In conventional Western medicine, this might be comparable to the vascular irregularities and vessel dilation that occur with a migraine attack.)

- Wind may cause our pain to shift from the temporal area to the back or the crown of our head (a forehead headache is usually related to the spleen-stomach pancreas network, the crown and back of the head to the kidney-bladder network, and the side or temporal area to the liver-gall bladder network).

- Dampness may cause our headache to have a heavy or oppressive feeling.

- Cold may make our headache worsen when the temperature drops.

- *Liver fire* is an extreme manifestation of stagnation of liver chi and excessive liver energy. When the energy flares up and rises to our head, besides causing a headache, it may overload our senses and irritate our cranial nerves, thus causing many of the other symptoms we experience such as visual, olfactory, and auditory auras, as well as dizziness, nausea, and vomiting. (In conventional Western medicine, this might be comparable to the cortical spreading depression theory, where a wave of hyperexcitability is thought to spread across the outer layer of the brain, irritate the cranial nerve roots, and cause many of these same symptoms.)

Kidney-Bladder Organ Network System

In TCM, any disorder or disease that affects the body can weaken the kidney-bladder organ network system. Prolonged disorders or illnesses can be extremely harmful. Thus, those of us with a long history of migraine disease, or chronic migraine, may find ourselves with a depletion in energy of the kidney-bladder network system:

- A deficiency in kidney energy allows fire to build up in our body, including our liver and our heart.

- The excess liver fire surges to our head and causes pain (in the heart, it may cause rapid heart rates and palpitations).

- Also, because the kidney is believed to be the controller of the adrenal glands and therefore determines overall life force, severe depletion of kidney energy is thought to cause adrenal crisis (in conventional Western medicine, severe stress, including long-term and chronic illness, is thought to cause depletion of the stress hormones secreted by the adrenal glands and lead to adrenal crisis. For those of us with migraine disease, depletion of our stress hormones can lead to chronic migraine).

Spleen-Pancreas-Stomach Network System

An excessive intake of sweet, greasy, or fatty foods, those rich in chemicals, dehydrogenated oils, MSG, preservatives, artificial sweeteners and high fructose corn syrup, as well as alcoholic beverages may produce damp phlegm or mucous. The damp phlegm may block the free flow of chi and blood to our head.

(In conventional Western medicine, alterations in serotonin levels are thought to cause an increase in cravings for rich and fatty foods, many of which are migraine triggers and can aggravate the sinus component of our attacks. See Chapter One for more information on serotonin and Chapter Three for more information on food triggers.)

Emotional Balancing and the Body, Mind, and Spirit Relationship

To begin with, let's look at the mind and spirit. In TCM, our mind and spirit are considered to be subtle states of energy. A balanced mind contributes to our feelings of self-worth, self-love, and self-respect. Our spirit is thought to be the essence of our being. Awareness of our own spirituality or self-awareness gives us inner peace. Prayer is a way for us to communicate our needs to whichever higher power we choose. If you believe in a higher power and pray for yourself or your loved ones to recover from illnesses, you're able to affect the nature of the universe and have positive results.

As well, positive thoughts are believed to attract positive energy, and negative thoughts are believed to attract negative energy. In health and illness, a focus on positive thoughts often enables us to overcome illness and have a successful recovery. In contrast, a focus on negative thoughts is more likely to end up with negative results.

Now, let's take a look at emotions. In TCM, emotions are thought to be a heavier form of energy. When they affect our mood in a positive way, they contribute to good health and wellness. When they affect our mood in a negative way, they can lead to poor health, chronic illnesses, and in our case, migraine attacks. Emotional balance is achieved through conscious awareness of our true feelings.

Dr. Mao has a *three-step* program he uses to guide his patients to a positive emotional life that has been crucial to my pursuit of wellness (see *Secrets of Self-Healing*, Avery, 2008), and that I have his permission to share with you. The three steps incorporate the emotional influences associated with the five elements and the organ network systems.

The *first step* is self-awareness. This step is more difficult than it sounds, as it requires you to be honest in acknowledging your true feelings. For example, I always considered myself to be a well-balanced, happy person. I blamed any emotional disturbances I experienced on a physical disorder or a personality trait. Irritability, frustration, and impatience were caused by my migraine attacks. Worry, fear, and anxiety were related to the shyness I experienced as a child (and which still haunts me today in new and strange situations). Hyperexcitability was a direct result of autonomic nervous system instability. And any other emotional outbursts were definitely hormonal.

Self-awareness came for me when I realized that my physical disorders were not responsible for my emotional imbalances. Rather, my emotional imbalances were part of a mind, spirit connection that often led to a physical disorder. For example, anger can be a healthy emotion. But, because I do not like confrontation, I tended to suppress the feeling. This caused me to clench my teeth and tense the muscles in my neck, shoulders, and jaw, which then precipitated a migraine attack. Because I did not want to think of myself as a perfectionist, I internalized feelings like worry and fear of failure, which tended to interrupt my sleep and again precipitated many of my migraine attacks. Because I did not accept responsibility for my driven personality, I ran on adrenalin (epinephrine), often eating the wrong food or not eating at all, until my fuel tank was empty. Then I crashed, which not only precipitated a migraine attack, but heart palpitations, extra heartbeats, and episodes of tachycardia.

The *second step* is to connect your emotional energies to the corresponding element. When I first saw Dr. Mao, unbeknown to me, I suffered from a severe stagnation of liver energy, excessive liver fire, an enormous depletion in kidney energy that had catapulted me into adrenal crisis, and a problem with damp phlegm. However, now that I have learned to balance my emotions by expressing, or in some instances curbing, my feelings in a healthy way, my organ-network systems have become more stable.

For example, instead of repressing anger, I have given myself permission to tell someone, including my husband, that I am angry, irritable, or frustrated. This allows me to vent the emotion and let a constructive discussion ensue. If I am afraid or worried, I confront the cause rather than retreat inside and dwell on my inhibitions. When I am wired or riding high on joy and enthusiasm, I use meditation to calm me down.

The *third step* is to convert your emotional energy to health-enhancing energy. Balancing my emotional energy has allowed me to sleep better because I don't wake up in the night like I used to with a thousand things on my mind to torment me. Since I no longer run on adrenalin and live with a stomach tied up in knots, I eat more regular and nourishing meals. Because I am well rested and well nourished, I have increased my physical energy and am able to commit to a regular exercise program. In addition, my newfound energy has allowed me to take on new ventures such as healing touch therapy, which has given me tremendous spiritual gratification (see Chapter Nine for more information).

At this point, it is interesting to note that in conventional Western medicine, Holistic Medicine, and other types of Wellness Medicine, prayer, positive attitudes and effective coping mechanisms have proven to be effective in the management of stress, illness, and the pursuit of good health.

How Migraine Disease Is Diagnosed

Although TCM promotes the concept of wellness and taking care of yourself before a problem arises, it doesn't discourage regular appointments with your medical doctor and the importance of a correct medical diagnosis, including invasive procedures, to determine the cause of illness or disease. In Chapter Two, we looked at the importance of a correct medical diagnosis for migraine disease.

For the remainder of this chapter, we will look at how doctors of TCM diagnose migraine disease. If you recall, I told you that in my first appointment, after a lengthy interview with Dr. Mao, he took me to a treatment room, grasped both of my wrists and pressed his fingers to my pulse points, looked into my eyes, and asked me to stick out my tongue.

In TCM, diagnoses of disturbances in the organ network systems, including those involved with migraine disease, are detected through the practitioner's evaluation of what he or she hears, sees, smells, and feels.

Questions (Asking)

A comprehensive interview helps the practitioner determine the nature of the disorder, as well as a holistic picture of the patient. Questions you might expect to be asked may include those related to:

- Your past and present medical problems (physical, emotional, and mental)

- Your family history of physical, emotional, and mental disorders

- The presence and characteristics of your pain

- Your bowel and bladder function

- Any problems you have with heat or cold

- Any problems with thirst and appetite

- Any problems with weight loss or gain

- Your diet and eating habits

- Your hobbies, relaxation practices, and exercise routines

- Your work and home environments

- Your emotional health

- Your response to stress

Observations (Looking, Hearing, and Smelling)

In general, you're considered to be in good health if you have a sparkle in your eyes, a straight spine, are quick to respond to questions during your interview, your breath is fresh, voice strong, and speech clear. If your eyes are dull, shoulders slumped, and you have body odors, a weak voice, muffled speech, the presence of a cough, or a sluggish response, these are indicators to your doctor that you have disharmony and imbalance in one or more of your organ network systems.

More specific indicators of disturbances in the organ network systems are revealed through your doctor's inspection of your eyes, skin (complexion), tongue, palms, fingers, and nails. Each of these is divided into zones that reflect the five elements and the corresponding organ network systems (see Tables 7.1, 7.2, 7.3, 7.4, and 7.5, respectively).

The Eyes

The eyes are considered to be the windows of your soul. If you look into the eyes of others, you can assess the clarity of their spirit.

TABLE 7.1: ZONES OF THE EYES RELATED TO THE FIVE ELEMENTS AND THE CORRESPONDING ORGAN NETWORK SYSTEMS		
ZONE	ELEMENT	ONS
Whites	Metal	Lung–Large Intestine
Pupils	Water	Kidney–Bladder
Iris	Wood	Liver–Gall Bladder
Corners	Fire	Heart–Small Intestine
Eyelids	Earth	Spleen–Pancreas–Stomach

If you look into your own eyes, you may be able to detect signs of disease. For example, when the whites of your eyes are red, it may indicate allergies and/or disturbances in your lung-large intestine network. A yellow color may indicate a disorder in your liver-gall bladder network. A black or dark gray color around your eyes may represent a lack of sleep or, as in my case, a severe kidney deficiency and prolonged stasis of blood and chi related to an excess of fire energy.

The Face

A lustrous complexion with normal color indicates that you have ample chi and blood flow. A white or pale color may be a sign of chi or blood deficiency. A yellow color may indicate spleen deficiency and the accumulation of damp phlegm or a disturbance in your liver-gall bladder network. A red color reflects dilated blood vessels due to excessive heat. A blue color represents stasis

TABLE 7.2: ZONES OF THE FACE RELATED TO THE FIVE ELEMENTS AND THE CORRESPONDING ORGAN NETWORK SYSTEMS		
ZONE	**ELEMENT**	**ONS**
Forehead	Fire	Heart–Small Intestine
Nose	Earth	Spleen–Pancreas–Stomach
Right cheek	Metal	Lung–Large Intestine
Left cheek	Wood	Liver–Gall Bladder
Chin	Water	Kidney–Bladder

of blood and chi. And a gray or black color is indicative of severe kidney deficiency.

Changes in color, tone, blemishes, broken capillaries, and dark patches in a specific zone may also be indicative of a disorder in that organ network system. For example, pimples or redness on the tip or sides of your nose may indicate an imbalance in your earth element or spleen-pancreas-stomach network related to a diet high in spicy, fatty, or rich foods, including chocolate. Broken capillaries and redness in your left cheek may be a sign of excessive liver heat and congestion.

The Tongue

A healthy tongue should be pink and muscular, without tooth marks or coating. A red tongue indicates increased heat in your body. A deep red tongue is indicative of excessive heat or fire. A

TABLE 7.3: ZONES OF THE TONGUE RELATED TO THE FIVE ELEMENTS AND THE CORRESPONDING ORGAN NETWORK SYSTEMS

ZONE	ELEMENT	ONS
Tip	Fire	Heart–Small Intestine
Band-like area behind tip	Metal	Lung–Large Intestine
Right and left sides	Wood	Liver–Gall Bladder
Center	Earth	Spleen–Pancreas-Stomach
Back	Water	Kidney–Bladder

deep red tongue with red dots on the tip may reflect a disorder of your heart-small intestine network related to stress and tension.

Teeth marks on the sides of your tongue may be indicative of a disorder in your liver-gall bladder network. A thick white coat may indicate spleen deficiency. A thick yellow coat may be reflective of accumulation of heat in your body related to infection and inflammation. A half yellow and half white tongue may indicate accumulation of heat in your liver-gall bladder organ network system. A brown, gray, or sometimes black coating may indicate excess internal heat and a scorching of body fluids. A tongue that looks like spots were scraped out from certain areas may indicate a disorder in the corresponding organ-network system.

The Palms

Disorders of the organ network systems can be revealed through the color, peeling, swelling, hardness, or itchiness of the

TABLE 7.4: ZONES OF THE PALMS OF THE HANDS RELATED TO THE FIVE ELEMENTS AND THE CORRESPONDING ORGAN NETWORK SYSTEMS		
ZONE	ELEMENT	ONS
Under third finger to right of middle of palm	Fire	Heart–Small Intestine
Upper portion of palm under index finger	Wood	Liver–Gall Bladder
Fleshy part of palm below thumb	Metal	Lung–Large Intestine
Portion beneath fourth and fifth fingers, including sides of hand and upper two-thirds of palm	Earth	Spleen–Pancreas–Stomach
Fleshy part beneath earth zone and above wrist	Water	Kidney–Bladder

connected zone. For example, disorders of your kidney-bladder network system may be reflected through swelling, or a purplish discoloration, in the water element.

The Fingers and Nails

Dry skin and redness may reflect heat or hyperactivity in the corresponding network system. Swelling or nodules may indicate a blockage in energy flow (chi). The sheen, quality, and texture of the skin behind your nails, as well as ridges and markings, may reflect a deficiency in the appropriate organ network system.

TABLE 7.5: FINGERS RELATED TO THE FIVE ELEMENTS AND THE CORRESPONDING ORGAN NETWORK SYSTEMS		
ZONE	**ELEMENT**	**ONS**
Thumb	Metal	Lung–Large Intestine
Index finger	Wood	Liver–Gall Bladder
Middle finger	Fire	Heart–Small Intestine
Ring finger	Water	Kidney–Bladder
Little finger	Earth	Spleen–Pancreas–Stomach

The Pulse (Feeling)

The pulses at your wrist provide valuable information for the TCM practitioner. Besides strength, regularity, and quality, there are numerous intricate waves that reflect disorders in the organ-network systems. In those of us with migraine disease, some of these may include

- A wiry pulse accompanied by a one-sided headache related to liver stagnation

- A wiry, forceful pulse accompanied by dizziness, ringing in our ears, and temporal headaches related to an excess of liver energy

- A wiry, forceful pulse accompanied by a red face, eyes, and tongue; thirst; irritability; insomnia; and a pulsating headache that may worsen with exercise and emotional stress related to flaring up of liver fire

- A choppy pulse accompanied by spots on our tongue and a fixed point of head pain related to blood stasis

- A weak pulse accompanied by fatigue, a pale tongue, and a headache of mild to moderate intensity related to kidney deficiency

- A slippery pulse accompanied by a thick coating on the tongue and a headache with a heavy sensation related to accumulation of damp phlegm

Looking Back and Glimpsing Ahead

In this chapter, you read that in TCM, migraine disease is looked at like any other disease, a disorder of the body as a whole. You discovered that the most common organ systems associated with migraine disease are the liver-gallbladder, kidney-bladder, and spleen-pancreas-stomach networks.

You also learned about emotions and the body, mind, spirit relationship. And you found out how emotions can be the cause of damage to our organ systems. When they affect us in a negative way, we remain receptive hosts for the invasion of other pathogens—and hence migraine attacks. To balance my emotions and decrease the damage to my organ systems, Dr. Mao guided me through a three-step program, which I shared with you so that you can apply it to yourself.

In this chapter, you also discovered that, in TCM, disturbances in the organ network systems, including those involved with migraine headaches, are detected through the practitioner's evaluation of what he or she hears, sees, smells, and feels. When imbalances are identified, corrective measures are taken to prevent disease.

As you become more familiar with the practice of TCM, you will be able to identify some of these imbalances yourself. For example, almost every morning, I stand in front of the mirror and check myself out. First, I look at my complexion, next I check out my eyes, and then I stick out my tongue and examine it for coatings and spots. My quick exam also helps me police my triggers. If I have changes in an area reflective of an organ system, I know I'm off course somewhere. Thus, I have to be more diligent about what I eat and drink and the measures I take to balance my emotions and manage the stress in my life. Otherwise, I am in for a migraine attack.

CHAPTER EIGHT

How TCM Treats Migraine Disease

In TCM, the treatment of migraine disease, like any other disorder, focuses on the adjustment of yin and yang energies and the regulation of the smooth flow of chi, blood, and moisture in the organ network systems involved. Now you know that the organ systems primarily associated with migraine disease include the liver-gallbladder, kidney-bladder, and spleen-pancreas-stomach networks, so we can look at therapy.

In TCM, therapy is customized to fit the individual. A wellness plan for migraine disease may include a combination of diet, herbs, techniques like acupuncture, acupressure, InfiniChi, Chinese therapeutic massage (Tui Na), mind-body exercises like tai chi and Qi Gong, and meditation.

The Role of Diet

To begin with, let's look at some general information about diet. Foods are thought to play a significant role in the yin/yang nature of the body. Along with nourishment, they are believed to affect the balance of energy. For example, warming foods have a stimulating effect, while cooling foods have a calming effect.

The selection of foods is based on the individual's need to bring about an optimum state of wellness. For example, if you're tired, sluggish, or depressed and tend to get chilled easily, the consumption of warm foods may increase your energy. On the other hand, if you tend to be hyperactive and get overheated, cooling foods may be more appropriate for you.

To assist in selection, foods are categorized into hot and warming, cold and cooling, and neutral. Foods like poultry, meats, eggs, and dairy are thought to be warming. Fruits, vegetables, and liquids are believed to be cooling. And other foods like fish, whole grains, beans, legumes, nuts, and seeds are believed to be neutral.

Now let's apply this information to migraine disease. For those of us who suffer from migraine headaches, warming foods may increase our liver heat and the flare up of liver fire. Rich, greasy, and fatty foods may lead to a sluggish digestive system, deficiency in our spleen-pancreas-stomach network, and the accumulation of damp phlegm.

Foods for us to avoid include hot, spicy foods, processed foods, refined foods such as white flour and sugar, preservatives, additives, MSG, fermented foods and beverages like vinegar and alcohol, artificial colors and sweeteners, high fructose corn syrup, soda, hydrogenated oils, red meat, pork, eggs, dairy products, fatty and greasy foods, rich and creamy sauces, sweets, chocolate, coffee, bananas, avocados, tofu, and soy products. Foods to be incorporated include most cooling and neutral foods like fruits, vegetables, fish, beans, legumes, and whole grains.

You may recognize many of the preceding foods as triggers for your migraine attacks. For more detailed guidelines on foods and beverages to avoid, as well as those to include and promote balance and harmony in the body, mind, and spirit, see food and beverage triggers in Chapter Three.

Herbal Remedies Available to Treat Migraine Disease

Herbal medicine has been practiced for years in numerous cultures throughout the world. Studies have shown that some of these herbs may help to reduce the pain associated with our migraine attacks through anti-inflammatory actions by affecting blood flow to our brain and by promoting muscle relaxation and sedation. A few of these herbs may also help with nausea. For information about the most common ones that can be purchased OTC as tablets, capsules, gels, sprays, ointments, tinctures, elixirs, and teas, see Table 8.1.

It is important to note that because we're unique in the complexity and symptoms of our disease, while one OTC herbal remedy may work for one person, it may not work for another. As well, to avoid side effects, you should not exceed the dose or frequency of administration recommended on the label. In addition, you should ensure that the herbs you take are distributed by a reputable source.

Herbal Supplements Your TCM Practitioner May Prescribe

Chinese herbs are classified as balancing, cleansing, or regenerating tonics, medicinal herbs, and potent medicinal herbs. Tonic herbs are used to support organ network functioning and prevent imbalances. Medicinal herbs are used to correct organ network imbalances and alleviate illnesses. Potent medicinal herbs are powerful healing agents and are used by licensed practitioners to treat more serious diseases.

Herbs are seldom used in isolation. A licensed TCM practitioner may combine a multitude of ingredients into a formula unique to the individual. You need to be aware, because these formulas vary with each person and their diagnosis and symptoms, that they cannot be transferred from one person to

TABLE 8.1: COMMON OTC HERBS AND THEIR ACTIONS, SIDE EFFECTS, AND PRECAUTIONS	
HERB	**ACTION, SIDE EFFECTS, AND PRECAUTIONS**
Butterbur (*Petasites hybridus*)	Thought to have anti-inflammatory properties. Believed to have an effect on vessel spasm and blood flow to the brain. Side effects may include headache, indigestion, fatigue, nausea and vomiting, constipation, or diarrhea. Should not be used if you're pregnant, nursing, or have liver or kidney disease (may cause liver damage) without your doctor's approval.
Feverfew (*Tancetum parthenium*)	Believed to have anti-inflammatory properties. Thought to inhibit platelet clumping (blood clotting), influence serotonin levels, and affect vessel tone. Side effects may include abdominal pain, gas, nausea and vomiting, diarrhea, and nervousness. May increase bleeding times, so should not be taken with other blood thinning herbs and medications such as aspirin and Coumadin without your physician's approval.
Ginkgo biloba	Thought to inhibit platelet clumping and affect blood flow to the brain. May also have anti-inflammatory properties. Side effects may include dizziness, upset stomach, diarrhea, mouth sores, or irritation around the mouth. May affect insulin and blood sugar levels, so should not be taken by diabetics without doctor's approval. Like feverfew, should not be taken with other blood thinning herbs and medications without your doctor's approval.

TABLE 8.1: COMMON OTC HERBS AND THEIR ACTIONS, SIDE EFFECTS, AND PRECAUTIONS	
HERB	**ACTION, SIDE EFFECTS, AND PRECAUTIONS**
White willow bark (*Salix alba*)	An analgesic with anti-inflammatory properties similar to aspirin. Side effects are similar to aspirin and include stomach upset, ulcers, bleeding, ringing in the ears, and inflammation of the kidney. Should not be taken with other analgesics or non-steroidal anti-inflammatory drugs, without your doctor's approval. Should not be taken with other drugs, or herbs, with blood thinning properties without your doctor's approval. May make beta blockers and diuretics less effective. May increase blood levels of phenytoin (Dilantin). Should not be taken if you're allergic to aspirin. Should not be given to children as they may develop Reye's syndrome (a disorder that damages the liver and the brain).
Turmeric (*Circuma longa*)	Thought to have anti-inflammatory properties. Thought to inhibit platelet clumping and affect blood flow to the brain. Should not be taken with any other blood thinning herbs and medications without your doctor's approval.
Ginger (*Gan Jiang*)	Is a calming herb with anti-inflammatory properties like aspirin. May inhibit platelet clumping and affect blood flow to the brain. Thought to help with the nausea associated with migraine headaches.

TABLE 8.1: COMMON OTC HERBS AND THEIR ACTIONS, SIDE EFFECTS, AND PRECAUTIONS	
HERB	**ACTION, SIDE EFFECTS, AND PRECAUTIONS**
Cayenne (*Capsicum frutescens*)	The main ingredient, capsaicin, is believed to have anti-inflammatory properties that may interfere with substance P (refer to Chapter One). Thought to affect blood flow to the brain.
Peppermint (*Mentha piperita*)	Is a calming herb with anti-inflammatory properties. Is also a nasal decongestant and may relieve the sinus congestion associated with migraine headaches. May help with nausea and vomiting associated with migraine headaches.
Gelstat Migraine	Is a mixture of feverfew and ginger (see above for actions and precautions associated with feverfew and ginger). Is available in a sublingual gel form, so is quick to absorb.
MigraSpray	Is a feverfew preparation that is sprayed under the tongue (see above for actions and precautions associated with feverfew).
MigreLief	Is a combination of feverfew, riboflavin (vitamin B2), and magnesium (see above for actions and precautions associated with feverfew, and refer to Chapter Three for more information on magnesium).
Lemon balm (*Melissa officinalis*), Valerian (*Valeriana officinalis*), and Skull cap (*Scutellaria lateriflora*)	Thought to help muscle relaxation and sedation. Should not be taken with prescribed narcotic analgesics, muscle relaxants, sedatives, or other CNS depressants without your doctor's permission.

another. In fact, a combination of herbs that do not match your diagnosis and symptoms can be harmful.

Customized blends of herbs for migraine disease target the external influences we looked at like wind, heat, damp, and cold, as well as internal imbalances we might have such as liver stagnation, kidney deficiency, and blood stasis. Examples of herbs that may be used in individualized formulas to treat migraine disease include *Chrysanthemum* (Ju hua), *Actractylodis* (Bai zhi), *Duhuo radix* (Du huo), *Shizonepetae* (Jing jie), *Ledebouriellae* (Fang feng), *Bupleurum chinnensis* (Chai hu), *Angelica sinensis* (Dong quai), *Paeonia lactiflora* (Bai shao), *Uncariae* (Gou teng), and *Gastrodiae* (Tian ma).

Raw herbs may be boiled or ground into powder and taken as tea. Ground herbs may also be swallowed as capsules and tablets or used in the form of tinctures, elixirs, and ointments. I take one mix of herbs prescribed by Dr. Mao as a tea, and two blends in capsule form.

Note that, because herbal therapy may be initiated while you continue to take medication, to avoid interactions, your TCM practitioner should be aware of all OTC and prescription medications, herbs, and supplements you're taking. Likewise, your doctor or other healthcare provider should be aware of all herbs, OTC or prescribed, you're taking, because many of these may interfere with prescription medications and other supplements, as well as cause bleeding or other side effects.

As well, you need to be aware that any herbs that affect blood clotting are usually discontinued at least two weeks prior to surgery or any other invasive procedure that may cause bleeding, such as extensive dental work. Consult with your doctor if you have a question. And a reminder: If you're pregnant or a nursing mother, you should not take any drugs, herbs, or supplements without the consent of your doctor.

What Is Acupuncture?

To begin with, let's review some information about the flow of energy in the body. As I discuss in Chapter Five, chi is the vital energy force that flows through our body and connects our organ network systems through channels known as meridians. There are twelve main channels that correspond to our organ network systems and through which energy is transferred. In addition, there are eight extraordinary channels that store, or provide, excess energy from the kidney network as needed. These twenty channels intersect, empty into one another, and connect the front of our body to the back, and the interior to the exterior.

The flow of chi through these channels is continuous. In general, yin energy, which corresponds to the front of our body, flows downward toward our back. Likewise, yang energy, which corresponds to the back of our body, flows upward toward our chest. When the flow of chi is disrupted, the involved channels become blocked and illness occurs.

Now let's apply this information to acupuncture. Acupuncture is a modality of TCM in which thin metal needles are inserted into sensitive points (also known as *gateways*) along blocked channels to reestablish the flow of chi and allow our body's self-healing mechanisms to occur.

There are twelve main and two minor groups of sensitive points. They are connected by lines, or pathways, that run from the top of our head to the tips of our fingers and toes. The placement of needles in sensitive points along these pathways is determined by our individual diagnosis, organ network system(s) affected, and associated symptoms.

How Acupuncture Works

As I mentioned, acupuncture clears blocked channels, balances the flow of chi, and allows for self-healing to occur. While accomplishing these functions, acupuncture:

- Eases pain and promotes relaxation by increasing the production of endorphins (natural pain killers).

- Decreases inflammation by increasing our body's production of natural corticosteroids.

- Balances our autonomic nervous system (sympathetic and parasympathetic branches) and our body's response to internal and external influences (many of which we know as triggers for our migraine attacks).

How Acupuncture Works for Migraine Disease

Along with the preceding effects, acupuncture is thought to:

- Balance our serotonin levels and help regulate blood flow in narrowed blood vessels.

- Reduce congestion in our head and redistribute chi and blood flow to our cold hands and feet.

- Relax tense muscles, relieve pain, and promote a feeling of well-being through an increase in our endorphin levels.

- Decrease the severity and frequency of our attacks by balancing our body's homeostatic response to internal and external stress (refer to Chapter Three for information about the stress response).

As I mentioned at the beginning of Chapter Five, the sessions last about an hour and involve minimal discomfort. You may feel a needle prick sensation at the site of insertion, or warmth, an ache, and numbness along the involved pathway. In general though, the sessions promote a feeling of relaxation and drowsiness. I often sleep through the procedure, and although I have needles in my head, face, neck, abdomen, hands, fingers, legs, and feet, I'm not aware of their presence.

The frequency of treatments varies with the response of the individual. In some instances, the response may be immediate. However, if you have suffered from migraine disease for a long period of time, it may take weeks or months of sessions at regular intervals before you see a profound effect.

In my case, although the severity of the attacks began to diminish after the first few treatments, it took several treatments before I noticed a distinct decrease in the number of attacks. Now, even though my migraines are rare, I continue to have acupuncture every six to eight weeks to keep my body in balance and prevent recurrence.

It is interesting to note that studies have shown that patients with migraine attacks respond very well to acupuncture. The response is even better when our treatments are complemented by changes in our diet, herbal therapies, stress reduction techniques, and moderate exercise.

Acupressure and How It Works for Migraine Disease

Acupressure uses finger or thumb pressure, rather than needles, to open blocked channels, restore the flow of chi, and promote self-healing. Common sites used to relieve migraine headaches at the onset include

- The valley of harmony, which is located on the web-bing between the thumb and index finger of both hands:
  - Using the thumb of one hand, press on this point until you feel soreness.

- Hold for two minutes and then repeat with the other thumb and hand.

- The Greater Yang (Taiyang), which is located in the indentation of the temples:

  - Massage the points with your knuckles, thumbs, or the tips of your index fingers in a circular motion for five minutes.

- The Wind Pond, which is located at the base of the skull in the natural indentation on both sides of the neck:

  - Press your thumbs on these points and lift upward towards your skull.

  - Lean your head back against your thumbs, and breathing evenly and regularly, maintain pressure for five minutes.

  - Use these points with caution, or avoid, if you have a neck or spinal injury, as manipulation may aggravate your condition.

InfiniChi and How It Helps Migraine Disease

InfiniChi is a Ni family (Dr Mao's) method of balancing energy in the body without the use of needles. Practitioners are trained to sense and manipulate energy with their hands. As the hands are held above the body and move downward from the head to the toes, weak areas are strengthened and excessive areas are purged. Light massage, acupressure, or guided visualization may be used to help direct the flow of energy.

The benefits of InfiniChi are similar to those of acupuncture and herbs. The treatment can be helpful in the treatment of migraines by redistributing the flow of energy from the head to the rest of the body.

Tui Na (Tuina) and How It Helps Migraine Disease

Tui Na is a Chinese therapeutic massage that has been practiced for thousands of years. Methods of the massage include those that specialize in soft tissue techniques, joint injuries, and muscle sprains. Some are similar to acupressure and focus on imbalances in the organ network systems and the depletion of energy, and others are thought to manipulate the musculoskeletal system and help with joint and nerve pain.

Tui Na can be used alone or in combination with herbal therapy and acupuncture. The practitioner uses the arms, hands, fingers, elbows, knees, and sometimes feet to open blocked energy channels, restore the flow of chi, and promote self-healing. The benefits are similar to those of acupuncture and acupressure. The treatment may be helpful in migraines, as an adjunct to acupuncture, by the restoration of the smooth flow of chi throughout the body.

Mind-Body Exercises

In TCM, mind-body exercises are rhythmic movements that engage the mind, body, and breath as one. The soft, slow, graceful, and deliberate movements promote balance of energy, optimal organ function, relaxation, and calmness. As the body is moving, the mind is trained to guide and redirect the flow of energy to reverse energy blockages, relieve congestion caused by chronic stress, and nourish nerves, muscles, and organs. Throughout the exercises, breathing is deep and uses the full capacity of the lungs to allow the maximum amount of oxygen to enter the bloodstream and reach the tissues.

Examples of these exercises include tai chi and Qi Gong. Tai chi is a continuous set of movements you complete in their entirety. Qi Gong is a short set of repetitive movements that can be learned at a faster pace (to see the "Harmony Tai Chi" instructional DVD and "Self-Healing Qi Gong" instructional DVD go to *www.askdrmao.com* and select Health Products).

There are many different styles of tai chi and Qi Gong. These are associated with a long history of varying family traditions in China, as well as a focus toward martial arts, healing, or spirituality (please see the "References" section at the end of the book for more detail on these).

How They Work for Migraine Disease

As I mention in Chapter Three, fast-paced and aggressive forms of exercise can deplete serotonin levels and propel the body into the "fight or flight" form of stress that can be harmful for those of us who suffer from migraine disease. On the other hand, slow and moderate types of exercise can increase our body's serotonin levels and promote calmness and relaxation.

Mind-body exercises such as the healing and spirituality forms of tai chi and Qi Gong can be especially beneficial to us as they:

- Restore balance to our affected organ network systems.

- Redistribute the congestion in our heads to our extremities.

- Provide more oxygen to our brain by using the full capacity of our lungs during the rhythmic movements.

- Turn off, or reset, our sympathetic nervous system response to stress and promote emotional balancing, relaxation, and calmness.

Meditation and How It's Helpful for Migraine Disease

Meditation has been practiced for thousands of years in numerous cultures throughout the world. The definitions of meditation are as varied as the forms of implementation. In general, whatever the technique, meditation is considered to be a contemplative act that quiets the mind and promotes relaxation and calmness.

In TCM, the relaxation induced is thought to open up energy channels and allow blood to circulate without obstruction through all the organ network systems. The body-mind connection is believed to help balance emotions. Emotional imbalance, as I have mentioned many times, is considered to be a major cause of disease.

Breathing is thought to be an essential part of meditation as it affects the autonomic nervous system and helps switch the more stressful sympathetic nervous system (fast) to the more relaxing parasympathetic nervous system (slow). Breathing deep into the "dan tien" area two inches directly below the navel (belly button) is believed to help cool down the fire energies in our body, strengthen our kidneys, and contribute to longevity.

For those of us who suffer from migraine disease, as I discuss in Chapter Three, chronic stress can drain our energy and lead to adrenal crisis. Meditation, coupled with deep abdominal breathing, can be helpful in regulating our response to stressful situations, as well as in aborting and preventing migraine attacks and strengthening our kidneys.

A simple visualization meditation I learned from Dr. Mao is called "White Light Meditation" (see *Secrets of Self-Healing*, Avery, 2008):

1. Sit or lie down in a comfortable position.

2. Close your eyes, clear your mind, and breathing deeply and slowly, picture a white light or clear mountain spring flow down to your abdomen.

3. As you exhale, visualize the white light, or water, run down from your abdomen to the soles of your feet and drain out.

Repeat the sequence for ten minutes and as often as necessary. I practice this meditation whenever I feel a tightness in my head, a change of pressure in my head, or sense a migraine on the horizon.

Another meditation I learned from Dr. Mao is a stress-release meditation (see the "Meditation for Stress Release" CD at *www.askdrmao.com;* select Health Products). I practice this meditation on a daily basis to maintain emotional balancing, and if I wake in the night and cannot go back to sleep because of an active mind:

1. Sit or lie down on your back in a comfortable position.

2. Close your eyes and breathe slowly and deeply into your abdomen, repeating the word "calm" with every exhalation.

3. Then, beginning at your temples and the sides of your face, breathe in and as you exhale say the word "calm" as you relax your facial muscles.

4. Repeat the procedure saying the word "calm" on every exhalation as you move down from the neck, shoulders, upper arms, elbows, forearms, wrists, hands, and fingers.

5. As you reach your fingers, visualize all the tension leaving your body through your finger tips.

6. When you're ready, breathe into your face and again repeat the word "calm" as you exhale.

7. Continue the sequence as you move down through your throat, chest, abdomen, thighs, knees, calves, ankles, and feet.

8. As you reach your feet, visualize all the tension leaving your body through your toes.

9. When you're ready, breathe into the crown and back of your head and once again repeat the word "calm" as you exhale.

10. Repeat this routine as you go from the back of your head to your neck, upper back, lower back, back of the thighs, calves, and heels.

11. When you reach your feet, picture all the tension leaving your body through the soles of your feet.

12. Return to your abdomen and breathing deeply into the "dan tien" position, rub one hand over your abdomen in a clockwise motion thirty-six times; then repeat in a counterclockwise motion for thirty-six times to restore energy.

13. When you're finished, rub the palms of your hands together until you feel heat; then place them over your eyes.

14. As the heat disappears, bring your hands down over your face.

It's interesting to note that numerous studies have shown meditation to be an effective tool in reducing stress, controlling blood pressure, and managing pain.

Looking Back and Glimpsing Ahead

In this chapter, you learned that in TCM, treatment of migraine disease focuses on the adjustment of yin-yang energies and the regulation of the smooth flow of chi, blood, and moisture in our liver-gallbladder, kidney-bladder, and spleen-pancreas-stomach networks. You discovered that therapy is customized to fit the individual and can include a combination of diet, herbs, acupuncture, acupressure, InfiniChi, therapeutic massage, mind-body exercises, and meditation.

Now let's apply this information to our wellness plans. First, take a look at mine:

- To balance my yin-yang energies and decrease my liver fire and the accumulation of damp phlegm:

    - I avoid hot and spicy foods, refined and processed foods, those with additives and preservatives, fermented foods, most dairy products, rich and creamy foods, fatty and greasy foods, and stimulants.

    - I eat a well-balanced diet of organic fish, chicken, fresh fruits and vegetables, whole grains, and a small amount of lean red meat, pork, cheese, and eggs.

- To open blocked channels in my body and promote the smooth flow of chi, and balance the sympathetic and parasympathetic branches of my nervous system, I have acupuncture treatments every six to eight weeks, which also help to relax tense muscles in my neck and shoulders, stabilize my serotonin levels, and relieve my pain by boosting my endorphin levels.

I talk about meditation and breathing exercises in the next chapter, but the important thing here is that I practice the meditations I've shared with you in this chapter on a daily basis to abort, and prevent, the frequency of my migraine attacks.

Now it's your turn. The first thing you need to do is ask yourself, "What do I do, apart from take medication or herbs, that helps me to reduce the frequency and severity of my migraine attacks?" If you have come up empty, you need to do some serious thinking about changing your diet, lifestyle, and stress reduction techniques.

On the other hand, if you have identified and made an effort to avoid your triggers, partake of a healthy diet that avoids most of the foods and beverages that increase liver fire and damp phlegm, and participate in a regular exercise program that doesn't deplete your adrenal hormones, you might want to consider incorporating some therapies like acupuncture, meditation and others, which I discuss in the next chapter, into your wellness plan.

PART THREE

Integrative Therapies

CHAPTER NINE

Integrative Therapies and How They Help with Migraine Attacks

As I MENTIONED IN the Introduction, and it's important for you to understand, integrative therapies are not alternatives to treatment that you choose because of a belief that conventional Western medicine doesn't meet your needs. Rather, you need to be aware that integrative therapies encompass a number of therapeutic options you can explore and combine with conventional Western medicine to enhance your personal pursuit of wellness.

Another thing for you to note is that many of the integrative therapies thought to be helpful in the treatment of migraine disease, and that we will look at in this chapter, have evolved from the philosophy of TCM. Because of their success, they have become more acceptable in the Western medical profession. Other treatments that we will examine have been part of Western medicine for many years.

The therapies we will look at in this chapter include physical therapy, chiropractic therapy, exercise, yoga, meditation, breathing techniques, biofeedback, cold therapy, massage, reflexology,

Reiki, and healing touch. A lengthy discussion of each of these practices is beyond the scope of this book. If you want more detailed information about a specific technique, please refer to the "References" section at the end of the book.

At this point, note that before you begin any of these treatments or practices, your diagnosis should be confirmed by your medical doctor. As I mention in Chapter Two, a discussion of your headache history and a thorough physical examination will help rule out any underlying organic cause for your headache, determine if you're suffering from more than one type of headache, and help provide an effective treatment plan for you. If you have a doctor who is resistant to integrative therapies, you may need to find one who is more receptive.

The Role of Physical Therapy

Physical therapy utilizes a number of noninvasive physical and electrical techniques to treat injuries and diseases that affect our muscles and joints. Physical therapy may be helpful in the treatment of migraines when our attacks are caused or aggravated by things such as:

- Injuries to our neck or cervical spine

- Muscle tension in our upper back and top of our neck

- Poor posture worsened by sitting for long periods in front of a computer or television

Treatments are targeted to relieve the pressure put on our nerves and blood vessels and stop pain from radiating up the back of our neck to our head and temples. Techniques may include exercises and physical activities to:

- Strengthen our muscles and decrease soft tissue damage around injured joints in our neck, shoulders, and spine.

- Restore mobility to our injured joints and prevent recurrence of injuries.

- Relieve muscle tension in our neck and shoulders.

- Correct poor posture.

In my situation, physical therapy has been instrumental in my path to wellness. After my neck injury, which I mention in an earlier chapter, my migraines boomed. My neurologist sent me to a chiropractor (see the upcoming section, "The Role of Chiropractic Therapy"). Because my neck was so wobbly, the chiropractor was reluctant to do anything but refer me to the physical therapist on his staff. The physical therapist taught me a sequence of exercises to strengthen the muscles in my neck.

When I began to feel better, I decided to begin an exercise program on my own and experimented with weights, yoga, and whatever else was in vogue at the moment. Consequently, I had an awful relapse, including a shoulder injury I reactivated that required surgery. As part of my rehabilitation, I was again referred to a physical therapist.

My first visit found my shoulders slumped, neck tipped back and mouth hanging wide open. A guided program that focused on correct posture (shoulders back and chest forward), cervical traction and neck stretching, as well as the best way to utilize a minimum amount of weights, helped get me back on track.

Today, I have full range of motion of my shoulder, and I am free of the muscle tension in my neck and upper back that had contributed to the frequency and severity of my migraine attacks. And I know never to initiate an exercise program of any kind without professional guidance.

The Role of Chiropractic Therapy

Chiropractic therapy originates from the theory that many diseases in the body come from misalignment of the vertebrae of the spine. The misalignment puts pressure on adjacent nerves and affects associated muscles and blood vessels. Manipulation of the spine and other structures is the preferred treatment.

When our migraine attacks are caused by misalignment of the vertebrae, chiropractic therapy is thought to provide relief through gentle stretching of our neck. The stretching realigns the vertebrae and eases pressure on our inflamed nerves. Treatments are also believed to help with muscle tension and restriction of movement in our neck, upper back, and shoulders related to stiff muscles and poor posture.

The Role of Exercise

A regular exercise routine helps maintain weight, good health, muscle tone, and circulation of blood throughout our body. Aerobic exercise, repeated about forty minutes at least three days a week, is also believed to reduce the effects of stress in a person's life.

For those of us who suffer from migraines, the type of exercise we choose may be significant in either reducing the frequency and severity of our migraine attacks or precipitating a migraine attack. Low- to moderate-intensity exercises such as walking and sports that rely on endurance rather than power like swimming, hiking, long-distance running, and tai chi can decrease the frequency and severity of our migraine attacks by:

- Increasing our serotonin levels

- Raising our endorphin levels (body's natural pain reliever)

- Helping in stress reduction by promoting a feeling of calmness and relaxation

Strenuous and high-intensity exercises, however, can precipitate or aggravate our migraine attacks because:

- Although they increase our endorphin levels, they also increase our epinephrine levels.

- The increase in our epinephrine levels may propel our body into the "fight or flight" stress response and decrease our serotonin levels.

- Some exercises, like heavy weight lifting, may cause muscle tightness or spasms in our upper body.

When we exercise is also important. If you feel a migraine coming on, a slow, short walk in the fresh air may provide relief. However, exercise during a full-blown migraine attack may be excruciatingly painful.

If fear of a migraine attack is keeping you sedentary, check with your doctor. A consultation with a qualified physical therapist or personal trainer may be what you need to plan and initiate an exercise program that is best for your situation.

For example, throughout my life, I have been competitive in sports. Whether it was high school track and field, volleyball, and basketball or tennis and half-marathons in my adult years, I had to win. At the end of every event, after I had pushed myself to the wall, I ended up in bed with a migraine. The competitive nature of the sport put not only physical stress on me but also emotional stress. However, now that I have learned to balance my emotions and avoid self-inflicted pressure, and with the guidance of some exceptional physical therapists, I am able to participate in the sports I enjoy and follow a moderate exercise program that has improved the quality of my life.

The Role of Yoga

Yoga is a mind-body practice of stretching, poses, breathing techniques, and meditation that originated in India thousands of years ago. There are many different types of yoga. Some focus on physical movements, postures, and breathing. Others are more oriented to meditation, wisdom, and spirituality (please see the "References" section at the end of the book for more detail).

The regular practice of yoga is believed to help increase flexibility, align vertebrae, strengthen muscles, nourish brain cells, rejuvenate organs, and assist with self-awareness and emotional balance. In particular, yoga is thought to benefit us by:

- Stretching out tense muscles in our back and neck

- Improving bad posture

- Helping to reduce our epinephrine levels by promoting a feeling of calmness and relaxation

At this point, it's important to note that postures that put pressure on our head, neck, and shoulders or any that are practiced incorrectly (as I found out) may trigger or worsen migraine attacks. Like any other exercise program, after checking with your doctor, it's best to contact a skilled professional to plan and implement a program that is best for you.

The Role of Meditation

In general, meditation is a contemplative act that quiets the mind and calms the body. The practice may be associated with religious traditions, spiritual concepts, and/or a focus on health and longevity. When coupled with deep abdominal breathing, meditation can be an effective way for us to promote relaxation and decrease the effects of stress in our body (see Chapter Eight and the "References" at the end of the book for more detailed discussions).

The Role of Breathing

For those of us who suffer from migraines, respirations (breaths) can become rapid and shallow because of stress, anxiety, and pain. Breathing exercises can help regulate our response to stressful situations, slow our respirations down, increase our oxygen intake, ease tense muscles, promote relaxation, and often abort our migraine attacks.

Breathing exercises are incorporated into almost every type of mind-body exercise, yoga, meditation, relaxation technique, and biofeedback. Some that can be practiced apart from these situations—whether you're sitting, lying, or standing—include rhythmic breathing, deep abdominal breathing, and guided imagery.

Rhythmic Breathing

Most of us are unaware of our breathing patterns. Rhythmic breathing involves inhaling and exhaling at a fixed pace while you pay attention to the flow of air going in and out of your body. The breath is not forced, and the chest and abdomen move as one unit. Some sources have you count to four or five as you inhale and exhale. I learned the technique long ago in nursing school and have stuck with the words "breathe in" and breathe out":

1. As you inhale slowly through your nose, say the words "breathe in."

2. As you exhale slowly through your nose or mouth, say the words "breathe out."

3. Concentrate on relaxing your muscles.

After you repeat the breaths a few times, you should start to feel calm.

Note that inhaling through your nose is necessary to warm, filter, and moisten the air you breathe. Exhaling through your mouth helps release any air that may be trapped in your chest (and is the preferred method of exhalation in many sports and lung disorders). Nose-breathing may be difficult if you have small nostrils, a deviated nasal septum, nasal congestion, sinus infection, allergies, or an injury.

Deep Abdominal Breathing

As I mention in Chapter Eight, deep abdominal breathing helps switch the more stressful sympathetic nervous system (fast) to the more relaxing parasympathetic nervous system (slow). When I first visited the migraine clinic, I learned this technique as belly-breathing:

1. Place your hands on your abdomen, fingers pointing toward each other and touching, about two inches below your navel.

2. Breathe deep into the area, and as your abdomen fills with air, feel your fingers slip away from contact.

3. As you slowly exhale, contract your abdomen and feel your fingers resume contact.

After a few breaths, you should begin to feel more relaxed.

Mental Imagery Relaxation

A focus on peaceful images in the mind is thought to create harmony between our mind and our body. When I first visited the migraine clinic, I learned this technique as guided imagery:

1. Create a peaceful place in your mind—for example, your favorite beach or vacation spot.

2. Breathe deep, but slow and in a regular rhythm.

3. As you inhale, concentrate on the air filling your lungs, chest, and abdomen.

4. As you exhale, let go of all negative thoughts and focus on positive affirmations like "I am strong, healthy, and free of pain."

After you repeat the pattern a few times, you should feel any tension leave your body.

The Role of Biofeedback

Biofeedback is a body-mind connection geared toward helping people consciously control their pulse, blood flow, muscle tension, and oxygen intake to increase relaxation, reduce stress, and relieve pain. A person may be hooked up to electronic sensors to help measure progress.

For those of us who suffer from migraines, biofeedback is believed to help redirect blood from the dilated arteries in our head to our cold hands and feet. The redistribution of blood flow is thought to relieve the throbbing and pulsating pain associated with our migraine attacks.

Here's a variation of a biofeedback exercise I learned at the migraine clinic, and which I continue to practice, especially if I feel a migraine attack on the horizon:

1. Assume a comfortable position, sitting or lying. (If you choose, have soothing or calming music playing in the background.)

2. Close your eyes and take slow, regular breaths.

3. As you breathe, say to yourself slowly and rhythmically:

My hands are heavy and warm.
My elbows are heavy and relaxed.
My shoulders are heavy and relaxed.
My forehead is cool and smooth.
My jaw is gentle and firm.
My head is heavy and relaxed.
My neck is heavy and relaxed.
My shoulders are heavy and relaxed.
My heartbeat is steady and slow.
My breathing is deep and even.
My abdomen is heavy and warm.
My hips are heavy and relaxed.
My legs are heavy and relaxed.
My ankles are heavy and loose.
My feet are heavy and warm.
I am relaxed and free of pain.

4. Relax and collapse; collapse and let go.

Repeat each phrase twice if necessary. When you finish, your hands and feet should feel warm, and you should feel drowsy and close to pain free.

The Role of Cold Therapy

Cold therapy, or *cryotherapy,* is believed to help narrow dilated vessels, reduce inflammation in adjacent tissues, relieve pressure on affected nerves, decrease muscle spasm and muscle tension, and numb pain. Cold therapy may be used alone or along with heat therapy as a treatment for many conditions including athletic injuries, orthopedic surgeries, and migraine attacks.

I have used cold therapy to numb the pain of migraine attacks since childhood. Numerous times I've lain with ice bags or frozen gel bags that covered my eyes, top of my head, and the back of my neck. Although the frozen therapy was not effective in reducing the frequency of my migraine attacks, the cold provided a distraction from the pounding sensation that made me want to put my head through the wall. Along with meditation, breathing techniques, and biofeedback, it also worked to dim the pain until whatever medication I could swallow and keep down, inject, or inhale became effective.

Today, besides ice packs and frozen gel packs, which tend to slip off your head and get lost in your bedding or fall on the floor, there are options such as an Ice Pillow, Migra-Cap, and Icekap that not only stay cool for a long period of time but also stay in place. The Ice Pillow is designed to provide support to your head and neck while sleeping, and when the frozen gel pack is inserted, is thought to ease pain from pinched nerves, stiffness, or neck injuries. The Migra-Cap covers your head, neck, forehead, and eyes. When the gel packs are inserted, these areas are cooled, and light is blocked out. The Icekap covers your forehead, top of the head, and neck and leaves the eyes open so you can move around. A blend of peppermint and lavender essential oils that can be applied to the neck, base of the skull, or top of the head is included to help reduce anxiety and promote relaxation (for more information on any of these products, see the "References" section at the end of the book for their websites).

At this point, note that cold therapy should be discontinued after thirty minutes or if severe numbness occurs in the area of application. If you're pregnant, nursing, are diabetic, or have circulatory problems, you should be especially cautious. Cold or frozen ice packs and gel packs should not be applied directly to your skin.

The Role of Massage Therapy

Massage therapy has been practiced in various forms for many years in a variety of cultures. Techniques are numerous and may include the application of methods such as kneading, stroking, tapping, compression, and vibration to the soft tissues and muscle structure of the body. Depending on the type of massage, lotions, oils, or powders may be used to reduce friction between the therapist's hands and the client.

Massage therapy is believed to reduce pain and tightness in muscles, improve circulation and oxygen delivery to the tissues, remove lactic waste, increase flexibility and mobility in muscles and joints, relieve stress, and promote relaxation. In some practices—for example, TCM—massage is thought to restore the flow of energy in the body (refer to Chapter Eight for more detail).

Massage therapy has proven to be beneficial for many chronic health conditions, including migraine headaches. Along with pain relief and stress reduction, regular treatments may help us sleep better.

It's important to note that deep massage anywhere near your head during a migraine attack may worsen your pain. And a word of caution before you begin treatments: If you have any underlying medical conditions, you need to consult with your doctor before beginning treatment. For example, in general, massage is not recommended if you have heart disease, are prone to blood clots, have open wounds or infectious diseases, or if you have had recent surgery, chemotherapy, or radiation treatments. If you're pregnant, your treatments should be performed only by a therapist certified in pregnancy massage.

The Role of Reflexology

Reflexology is a form of massage therapy where the therapist applies pressure to reflex points, or *zones,* on the soles of the feet and the palms of the hands. Manipulation of these points with the hands, thumbs, or fingers is thought to:

- Open energy channels in the body.

- Send messages to correlating organs or parts of the body to correct imbalances.

- Assist the body with its innate ability to heal itself.

Reflexology techniques have proven to be effective in improving circulation, relieving pain, reducing stress, and promoting relaxation. For us, along with the techniques a reflexologist uses to reduce stress and promote relaxation, a qualified therapist may utilize specific techniques targeted to relieve pain and tension in our head, neck, and shoulders. Again, consult with your doctor if you have any underlying medical disorders or are pregnant.

The Role of Reiki

Reiki is an energy healing technique, which originated in Japan many years ago. The practice is based on the theory that life force flows around us in an energy field known as an aura, or *biofield,* and through us in pathways called meridians (refer to Chapter Five), energy channels are called *nadis,* and energy centers are referred to as *chakras.*

This life force, referred to as chi in TCM, is thought to nourish all the organs and cells of the body. As well, it is believed to be responsible for all of a person's thoughts and feelings. When our life force is disrupted or we have negative feelings about ourselves, functions of our organs and cells become diminished and disease and illness can occur.

The practice of Reiki is believed to restore the flow of life force and allow our body, mind, and spirit to heal itself. Benefits may include

- Stress reduction

- Relaxation

- Relief of aches and pains

- Clearance of toxins

- Increased immune function

- Acceleration of healing

- Increased self-awareness

- Spiritual growth

During a session, you can expect to be lying down and fully clothed. The practitioner's hands move above or gently touch your body in different locations. Energy is believed to channel from the universe through the practitioner's hands and then flow to wherever it is needed. A feeling of warmth is common among recipients. For those of us who suffer from migraines, Reiki treatments are believed to direct the flow of energy to correct our emotional imbalances, release tension, reduce the effects of stress, and promote relaxation.

The Role of Healing Touch

Healing touch is an energy-healing technique founded by Janet Mentgen, BS, RN, in the late 1980s. The practice is based on the theory that human beings are systems of energy. Energy flows from energy fields that surround the body (aura or biofield) to energy centers within the body (chakras) and is dispersed as necessary.

Blockages in this flow of energy are believed to have a profound effect on the physical, emotional, mental, and spiritual health of a person. The goal of healing touch is to open blocked energy centers (chakras), restore harmony and balance in the energy system, and assist the body to heal itself.

Success has been reported in a number of acute and chronic illnesses and disorders, including cancer, arthritis, multiple sclerosis, back and neck pain, headaches, and emotional disorders. Benefits are believed to include

- Decreased pain

- Reduction of anxiety, stress, tension, and depression

- Enhanced immune function

- Acceleration of recovery from surgical procedures

- Deepening spiritual connection

For those of us who suffer from migraines, healing touch is thought to relieve our headaches by opening our chakras, promoting relaxation, and stimulating the release of endorphins. As well, repeated treatments can help relieve tension in our neck and upper back that may contribute to the frequency and severity of our migraine attacks.

Like Reiki, during a session, you are lying down and fully clothed. You can expect a treatment to last anywhere from twenty to sixty minutes. In general, with your permission, the practitioner will begin by scanning your energy with the palms of his or her hands held above your body, moving from your head to your toes. Throughout your treatment, the practitioner's hands may be held above you or gently touch your body as he or she works to restore energy flow to the blocked or depleted areas detected. Like Reiki, you may experience a feeling of warmth as the practitioner's hands pass over your chakras, and you may even doze off during your treatment.

Since I have become involved with healing touch, whether giving a treatment to someone else or completing a session on myself, I've noticed an overwhelming sense of calmness and emotional stability. As I mention in Chapter Seven, balancing my emotional energy has played a huge role in decreasing the frequency and severity of my migraine attacks.

Looking Back and Glimpsing Ahead

In this chapter, you read about a number of integrative therapies that promote wellness by helping us to:

- Relax tense muscles in our neck and shoulders.

- Reduce muscle spasm and inflammation and relieve pressure on adjacent nerves.

- Balance our sympathetic and parasympathetic branches of our sympathetic nervous system and decrease the physical response of our bodies to stress (promote calmness and relaxation).

- Stabilize our serotonin levels.

- Increase our endorphin levels.

- Balance the flow of energy in our bodies.

- Increase self-awareness.

- Balance our emotions.

Note that while one of the integrative therapies we've looked at may be beneficial for one migraineur, it may not help another. The good news here is that there are a number of treatments you can pick and choose from to meet your particular needs.

As well, if one treatment is not available in your area—for example, healing touch—do not be discouraged. A similar one, like Reiki, might be within close proximity because many of these therapies are practiced in hospitals, long-term care facilities, spas, and wellness centers. And don't forget: After initial instruction in the technique, many of these therapies, such as meditation and breathing exercises, can be practiced in the comfort of your own home or office.

In addition, it's important for you to understand that the majority of these therapies have their greatest benefits over time, with sessions at regular intervals. And, like acupuncture, all of these therapies are more effective when they're combined with a healthy diet and lifestyle, which includes avoiding your identified triggers.

Now let's apply this information to our wellness plans. First, take a look at mine:

- To strengthen the muscles in my neck and prevent reoccurrence of my injury, every day I do the neck exercises I was taught by a physical therapist years ago.

- To increase my serotonin and endorphin levels, I walk four miles, three to four times a week, and follow a moderate exercise regime of weights and stretches that I learned from another physical therapist.

- To abort migraine attacks at the onset, I practice the deep breathing, biofeedback, and meditation techniques I have shared with you in these last two chapters.

- To numb the pain of a headache and decrease the associated inflammation, I use cold gel packs.

- To balance the energy centers in my body and increase self-awareness and spirituality, I practice the three steps I shared with you in Chapter Eight and healing touch.

- To reduce my body's physiological response to stress, increase my serotonin and endorphin levels, and promote emotional balancing, calmness and relaxation, along with exercise, deep breathing techniques, meditation, and healing touch, I have acupuncture treatments every six to eight weeks.

Now it's your turn. Following my guidelines, apart from medication and herbs, write down what you do, or plan to do, to abort, prevent, and manage your migraine attacks and to reduce your stress response. You will notice your answers will differ from mine. For example, you may not have a neck injury. Therefore, neck exercises may not be part of your wellness plan. As well, you may prefer yoga rather than walking for regular exercise. Or you may prefer Reiki over healing touch as an energy balancing therapy. Or you may find acupuncture, meditation, and a mind-body exercise like tai chi suit you just fine. The important thing here is that you choose some things that you can do on a regular basis to help you get well.

As you implement the integrative therapies you've chosen, document them along with their effects on the calendar you established in Chapter Three. It will take time, but if you stay committed, like me, you will see a reduction in the amount of medication you take and an increase in the amount of time you have to spend with your friends, family, and job.

PART FOUR

||||||||||||||||||||||||||||||||||||||||||||||||||||||||||||||||||||||||||||||||||||||||||||||||||||||||||||||||||||||||||||||

Your Journey

||||||||||||||||||||||||||||||||||||||||||||||||||||||||||||||||||||||||||||||||||||||||||||||||||||||||||||||||||||||||||||||

CHAPTER TEN

Guidelines to Help
You in Your Journey

IN THIS BOOK, YOU have learned what migraine disease is, where it comes from, and how it is diagnosed and treated in Western and Eastern medicine. You also discovered, through numerous techniques and therapies that I've shared with you from my personal wellness plan, how to develop your own self-care plan.

From this point on, your path to wellness is your own. The desire to achieve an optimal state of wellness is the beginning of your journey.

I will leave you with a few more suggestions and resources that you may find helpful to assist you on your way:

1. Pursue a sound body of knowledge.
We all want, especially in the throes of a violent attack, a magic pill or, even better, a life-long cure. Until medical research makes this information available and ensures the facts are reliable, our best hope is to arm ourselves with as much credible knowledge about the disease as possible. Some resources you may want to tap, include

MAGNUM (Migraine Awareness Group: a National Understanding for Migraineurs—*www.migraines.org*):

- Promotes migraine as a biologic, neurological disease.

- Offers support to sufferers, families, and coworkers.

- Offers up-to-date information about the disease and treatment options.

American Headache Society Committee for Headache Education (AHS—*www.americanheadachesociety.org*):

- Provides education for headache sufferers, migraineurs, and their families.

Migraine.com (*www.migraine.com*)

- Goal is to empower patients and caregivers to take control of migraine disease

- Provides a platform to learn, educate, and connect

Migraine Research Foundation (*www. migraineresearchfoundation.org*):

- Provides information about migraines to migraineurs.

- Raises money to promote research that contributes to the cause, understanding, and treatment of migraine.

American Migraine Foundation (*www. americanmigrainefoundation.org*):

- Offers information about migraines and promotes migraine research.

National Headache Foundation (NHF—*www. headaches.org*):

- Offers information for those who suffer from migraines and their friends and families.

2. Do your homework.

Migraine disease can be difficult to diagnose, especially if it's accompanied by a comorbid disease. If you're having difficulty in finding a doctor who is able to give you a definitive diagnosis, you may want to visit the Migraine Research Foundation's website for a list of doctors who are certified in Headache Medicine.

If you're interested in a holistic doctor, doctor of TCM, homeopathic doctor, naturopathic doctor, or any of the integrative therapies discussed in this book, you should ensure that any therapist or practitioner you choose is licensed or certified in his or her field. Resources you may want to utilize to find therapists or practitioners in your area, the cost of treatments, and whether they might be covered by your insurance, as well as credibility and levels of expertise of the provider, include

American Holistic Medical Association (AHMA— *www.holisticmedicine.org*):

- Serves as an advocate for the use of holistic and integrative medicine by all licensed healthcare providers.

American Integrative Medical Association (AIMA— *http://aihcp-norfolkva.org*):

- Is a professional certification and credentialing agency for medical practitioners of Integrative Medicine and Health Care.

- Mission is to enhance public trust in integrative medicine (complementary and alternative).

American Association of Integrative Medicine (AAIM—*www.aaimedicine.com*):

- Promotes the development of integrative medicine as the medicine of the 21st century.

American Holistic Nurses Association (AHNA—*www.ahna.org*):

- Is an association for nurses and other holistic healthcare professionals that promotes the education of nurses and other healthcare professionals and the public in aspects of holistic caring and healing.

Holistic Healing Web Page (*www.holisticmed.com*):

- Provides an extensive list of integrative therapies such as acupuncture, chiropractics, meditation, massage, and yoga and energy healing techniques like Reiki that you can go directly to or browse to find licensed or certified practitioners in your area.

Acupuncture.Com (*www.acupuncture.com*):

- A comprehensive site for information about acupuncture, acupressure, Chinese herbal medicine, nutrition, Tui Na bodywork, tai chi, Qi Gong, and related healing practices.

- Provides a directory of licensed practitioners throughout the United States.

Ask Dr. Mao: The Natural Health Search Engine (*www.askdrmao.com*):

- Site for all Dr. Mao's books and health products.

Healing Touch International (*www.healingtouchinternational.org*):

- Provides information about healing touch.

- Helps you find a certified healing touch practitioner near you.

Healing Touch Program (*www.healingtouchprogram.com*):

- Offers information about healing touch.

- Helps you find a certified healing touch practitioner near you.

Note that these resources are not offered to take the place of conventional Western medicine, but to assist you in your search for a qualified and credible therapist or practitioner who specializes in integrative therapies available in your area. Additional information on these sites, such as recommendations for supplements or other treatments, should be discussed with your doctor. As well, your doctor should be aware of any integrative program or treatment you want to start before you begin sessions or programs.

3. Create an environment conducive to wellness.
An environment conducive to wellness can flourish when balance and harmony exist within yourself (internal energies) and between yourself and your surroundings (external energies). Constructive principles include

- Identify, manage and, where possible, eliminate your personal triggers.

- If the list of food and beverage triggers in Chapter Three seems overwhelming, begin by eliminating the most popular triggers like chocolate, alcohol, caffeine, fast food, junk food, sodas, and anything with additives, preservatives, MSG, pesticides, herbicides, and antibiotics.

- While avoiding your individual triggers, eat organic produce, grains including cereals and breads, dairy products, meats, fish, and poultry whenever possible.

- Establish regular meal times as hypoglycemia can trigger an attack.

- Avoid fasting as, again, hypoglycemia can trigger an attack.

- Stay hydrated as dehydration can trigger an attack.

- Avoid environmental pollutants and toxins whenever you can.

- Use drugs, herbs, and supplements with discretion.

- Know the dosages, actions, side effects, and interactions of all drugs, herbs, and supplements you're taking.

- Follow the directions prescribed by your doctor or licensed practitioner to avoid rebound headaches and toxic reactions.

- Correct bad posture and reduce the strain on muscles in your neck and shoulders.

- Check with your doctor, and then begin a moderate exercise program to help regulate serotonin levels.

- Learn to balance your emotions and control your body's physiological response to perceived stressors through self-awareness, daily meditation, biofeedback, guided imagery, and similar focused-breathing techniques.

- Incorporate other integrative therapies such as acupuncture, mind-body exercises like tai chi, yoga, reflexology, Reiki, and healing touch into your wellness plan to help reduce the effects of stress, correct energy imbalances in your body, decrease the frequency and severity of migraine attacks, and limit your dependence on medication.

- If you're an overachiever, learn to set priorities, delegate, say "no," and keep a balance in your daily schedule so one activity does not impose on others.

- Maintain a regular sleep schedule as fatigue can trigger an attack.

4. Maintain a positive attitude.

Clear the clutter from your mind and focus on positive thoughts.

- Positive thoughts attract positive energy.

- A focus on positive thoughts and attitudes has been proven to help one have a successful recovery from illness—hence the phrases, "I have cancer, it does not have me," and in our situation, "I have migraine disease, it does not have me."

5. Enjoy the ride.

If you have had migraine attacks for years and, in particular, if you have consumed a load of medication and suffer from rebound headaches, expect that it will take some time to rid your system of toxins and allow any one of the integrative therapies discussed in this book a bit, if not a lot, of time to work.

When you have setbacks, concentrate on the good days when you are free of pain and the drugged sensation and hangover effect that medication gives isn't around. As times passes, with willingness and persistence, the good days will start to outnumber the bad days, and before you know it, you may, as I do, be saying to yourself, "When exactly was my last headache?"

Good luck and good health!

References

Alexander, D. (2008, April 8). "Treating Headaches with Physiotherapy." *GoToSee.co.uk.* Retrieved October 7, 2009, from *www.gotosee.co.uk*

Alexander, L., PhC. (2012). "Migraine—A Common and Distressing Disorder." *Headache Australia.* Retrieved December 10, 2012, from *www.headacheaustralia.org*

Allison, N., M.S., R.D., and C. Beck, M.S. *Full & Fulfilled: The Science of Eating to Your Soul's Satisfaction.* (Nashville, TN: AB Publishing, 1998, 2000).

American Council for Headache Education. (2000). "What's the Best Medicine for My Headaches?" *HealingWell.com LLC.* Retrieved November 20, 2010, from *www.healingwell.com*

The American Headache Society Committee on Headache Education (ACHE). (2011). "Migraine and Common Morbidities." Retrieved December 10, 2012, from *www. achenet.org*

Amoils, S., M.D., and S. Amoils, M.D. *Get Well & Stay Well.* (Ohio: Integrative Medicine Foundation, 2011).

Appel, S., M.D., et al. (2005, May 19). "Evidence for Instability of the Autonomic Nervous System in Patients with Migraine." *Headache: The Journal of Head and Face Pain.* Retrieved January 1, 2010, from *www3.interscience.wiley.com*

Bartley, J., and T. Clifton-Smith. "Breathing Patterns," from *Breathing Matters*. (Auckland, New Zealand: Random House, 2006).

Batliner, A., NC, Dipl. ABT, CST. (2004). "Liver Qi Stagnation and Diet." *Nutrition Professionals Quarterly.*

Beinfield, H., L.Ac., and E. Korngold, L.Ac., O.M.D. *Between Heaven and Earth: A Guide to Chinese Medicine.* (New York: Ballantine Books, 1991).

————"Traditional Chinese Medicine: Chinese Medicine: How It Works." *Looking for More Balance in Your Life?* Retrieved January 16, 2011, from *www.healthy.net*

Bernstein, C., M.D. *The Migraine Brain.* (New York: Free Press, 2008).

Biomed Central. (2006, September 28). "High Risk of Migraine, Depression and Chronic Pain for IBS Sufferers, Large Study Shows." *ScienceDaily.* Retrieved December 10, 2012, from *www.sciencedaily.com*

Blakeslee, S. (1996, January 23). "Complex and Hidden Brain in the Gut." *The New York Times.* Retrieved September 26, 2011, from *www.universal-tao.com*

Blaylock, R. L., M.D. *Excitotoxins.* (Albuquerque: Health Press, 1997).

———— ed. (2010). "Killer Headaches: Natural Ways to Stop and Prevent Them." *The Blaylock Wellness Report: Living a Long, Healthy Life, 7*(7): 1-10.

Block IV, E. F. (2011, February). "The Traditional Chinese Medicine Concept of Dampness." Retrieved March 3, 2011, from *www.diamondhead.net*

Boeree, C. G., Dr. (2009). "Neurotransmitters." *General Psychology.* Retrieved April 19, 2010, from *http://webspace.ship.edu*

Brennan, B. A. *Hands of Light: A Guide to Healing Through the Human Energy Field.* (New York: Bantam Books, 1988).

———. *Light Emerging: The Journey of Personal Healing.* (New York: Bantam Books, 1993).

Buchholz, D., M.D. *Heal Your Headache.* (New York: Workman Publishing Company, Inc., 2002).

Cady, R., M.D. (2007). "Pathophysiology of Migraine." *Pain Practitioner, 17*(1): 6–10.

Cady, R., and C. Schreiber. (2008). "Botulinum Toxin Type A as Migraine Preventive Treatment in Patients Previously Failing Oral Prophylactic Treatment Due to Compliance Issues." *Headache, 48*(6): 900–13.

Carter, B., MS., LAc. "Migraine Headaches: Medicines for Relief, Natural Treatments, Causes and Cures." Retrieved February 11, 2010, from *www.pulsemed.org*

Chawla, J., MBBS., MD., MBA., et al. (2011, May 25). "Migraine Headache." Retrieved January 7, 2013, from *www.emedicine.medscape.com*

Coleman, M. J., and T. M. Burchfield. "Migraines: Myth Vs. Reality." *MAGNUM.* Retrieved December 31, 2009, from *www.migraines.org*

De Vane, L. C. (2001). "Substance P: A New Era, a New Role." *Pharmacotherapy, 21*(9): 1061–9.

Dewitt-Carson, R. (2009, February 15). "Alternative Therapies for Treating Migraines." Retrieved December 12, 2012, from *www.headaches.about.com*

Diamond, S., M.D. (2011, January 1). "New Advances in Migraine Diagnosis and Treatment." *US DOCTOR.* Retrieved February 28, 2011, from *www.usdoctor.com*

Diamond, S., M.D., and M. A. Franklin. *Conquering Your Migraine.* (New York: Simon & Schuster, 2001).

Encyclopedia of Children's Health. "Narcotic Drugs." Retrieved December 10, 2012, from *www.healthofchildren.com*

Evans, R. W., M.D., C. Sun, M.D., and C. Lay, M.D. (2007). "Alcohol Hangover Headache." *The Journal of Head and Face Pain, 47*(2): 277–279.

Fear, B. (2005, November 16). "Biofeedback for the Treatment/ Prevention of Migraine Headaches." *Health Psychology Home Page.* Retrieved October 5, 2010, from *http://healthpsych.psy. vanderbilt.edu*

Ford-Martin, P. *The Everything Health Guide to Migraines.* (Avon, MA: Adams Media, an F&W Publications Company, 2008).

Gershon, Michael, M.D. *The Second Brain.* (New York: HarperCollins Publishers, 1998).

Gilbert, K. (2006, June 28). "Migraines and the Chiropractor's Touch." *Psychology Today.* Retrieved June 9, 2011, from *www. psychologytoday.com*

Goeway, D. J. *Mystic Cool.* (New York: Atria Books, 2009).

Hadhazy, A. (2010, February 12). "Think Twice: How the Gut's 'Second Brain' Influences Mood and Well-Being." *Scientific American.* Retrieved September 26, 2011, from *www.scientificamerican.com*

Hain, T. C., M.D. (2009, November 16). "IHS Criteria for Migraine." *Dizziness-and-balance.com.* Retrieved February 11, 2010, from *www.dizziness-and-balance.com*

Hart, C., Ph.D. *Secrets of Serotonin.* (Lynn Sonberg Book Associates, New York: St. Martin's Press, 2008).

"Headache, Migraine In-Depth Report." *The New York Times.* Retrieved November 27, 2010, from *http://healthnytimes.com*

Hiatt, K. (2010, October 21). "A New Route to Migraine Relief: Botox?" *US News and World Report.* Retrieved November 5, 2010, from *http://health.usnews.com*

Hoffman, R., M.D., CNS. "Mitral Valve Prolapse." *Dr. Ronald Hoffman*. Retrieved November 8, 2009, from *www.drhoffman.com*

Hover-Kramer, D., EdD., RN. *Healing Touch: A Guidebook for Practitioners* (2nd Edition). (Delmar, Cengage Learning, 2002).

Hutchinson, S. L., M.D., and S. J. Tepper, M.D. (2009). "Treatment and Management of Migraines—The Road Ahead." *US Neurology,* 5(1): 72–74.

International Headache Society. (2004). "The International Classification of Headache Disorders" (2nd Edition). *Cephalalgia, 24,* suppl 1: 9–160.

John, P. J., N. Sharma, C. M. Sharma, and A. Kankane. (2007). "Effectiveness of Yoga Therapy in the Treatment of Migraine Without Aura: A Randomized Controlled Trial." *Headache,* 47(5): 654–651.

Jones, A. "Home-Icekap." Retrieved June 9, 2011, from *www.icekap.ca*

Kister, I., et al. (2010). "Migraine Is Comorbid with Multiple Sclerosis and Associated with a More Symptomatic MS Course." *The Journal of Headache and Pain, 11*(5): 417–425.

Kumar, P. "Three Step Rhythmic Breathing." *Life Positive.* Retrieved June 23, 2011, from *www.lifepositive.com*

Kunz, B., and K. Kunz. "What Is Reflexology?" *Reflexology-Research.* Retrieved June 23, 2011, from *www.reflexology-research.com*

Lal, V., and M. Singla. (2010). "Migraine Comorbidities—A Discussion." *Supplement of JAPI, 4,* (58): 18–20.

Laverie, S. (2010, May 26). "Little-Known Herb Butterbur Cures Symptoms of Migraine Headaches." *sojustask.* Retrieved March 26, 2011, from *http://scam.com*

Mannix, L. K., M.D. (2004, September 1). "Comorbities of Migraine." *National Headache Foundation,* 1–8.

Martin, V. T., M.D." Menstrual Migraine: New Approaches to Diagnosis and Treatment." American Headache Society. Retrieved January 28, 2013, from *www.americanheadachesociety.org*

Martin, V., and A. Elkind. (2004). "Diagnosis and Classification of Primary Headache Disorders." In *Standards of Care for Headache Diagnosis and Treatment: National Headache Foundation.* (pp. 4–18). Chicago (IL).

Mauskop, A., M.D., and B. Fox, Ph.D. *What Your Doctor May Not Tell You About Migraines.* (New York: Wellness Central, 2001).

Mawe, G. M., T. A. Branchek, and M. D. Gershon. (1986). "Peripheral Neural Serotonin Receptors: Identification and Characterization with Specific Antagonists and Agonists." *Proc. Natl. Acad. Sci. USA, 83:* 9799–9803.

Mayo Clinic Staff. (2011, June 4). "Migraine: Treatments and Drugs." Retrieved December 10, 2012, from *www.mayoclinic.com*

McMillan, D. L., MA. (2000, September 16). "An Integrative Model of Migraine Based on Intestinal Etiology." *Meridian Institute.* Retrieved November 5, 2010, from *www.meridian-institute.com*

Migra Spray. *Spinelife.com.* Retrieved April 4, 2011, from *http://spinelife.stores.yahoo.net*

"Migraine Headache in Children Causes, Triggers, Types, Symptoms . . ." Retrieved December 10, 2012, from *www.emedicine-health.com*

Miles, O. (2010, November). "Cold Therapy." *Migraine.com.* Retrieved June 23, 2011, from *http://migraine.com*

———. (2010, November). "Gingko Biloba." *Migraine.com.* Retrieved March 29, 2011, from *http://migraine.com*

Miller, D. (2008, September 11). "What Does GABA Do in the Brain?" *Articlesbase.* Retrieved December 7, 2010, from *www.articlesbase.com*

Millichap, J. G., M.D., F.R.C.P. (2002). "The Role of Diet in Migraine Headaches." *NOHA NEWS, XXVII* (3): 3–6.

Mitchell, D. (2010, September 27). "Gene Called TRESK Causes Migraine, Controls Pain." *EmaxHealth.* Retrieved November 5, 2010, from *www.emaxhealth.com*

Moloney, M. E., PhD., RN, ANP-BC, and L. A. Cranwell-Bruce, MS, RN, FNP-BC. (2010). "Pharmacological Management of Migraine Headaches." *The Nurse Practitioner, 35*(9): 16–22.

National Headache Foundation. "Low Tyramine Diet for Migraine." Retrieved December 10, 2012, from *www.headaches.org*

Navia, J. (2002, January 8). "Could Tannins Explain Classic Migraine Triggers?" *Tannin Home.* Retrieved January 26, 2012, from *www.widowmaker.com*

Ni, M., L.Ac., D.O.M., PH.D. *Secrets of Self-Healing.* (New York: Avery, 2008).

Nicole, G. D., D. K. Klinberg, and M. R. Vasko. (1992). "Prostaglandin E2 Increases Calcium Conductance and Stimulates Release of Substance P in Avian Sensory Neurons." *Journal of Neuroscience, 12*: 1917–1927.

Pain Management Health Center. "Nonsteroidal Anti-Inflammatory Drugs (NSAIDs)." (2010, February 3). *WebMD.* Retrieved September 30, 2010, from *www.webmd.com*

———"Opioid Pain Relievers for Chronic Pain." (2011). Retrieved December 10, 2012, from *www.webmd.com*

Petersen, V., M.D., and R. Petersen, M.D., D.C., C.C.N. *The Gluten Effect.* (United States of America: True Health Publishing, 2009).

Ralston, Meredith. "Migraine: The Result of a Misunderstood Chemical Reaction Involving Neurotransmitters and Vasoamines." Retrieved December 10, 2012, from *www.serendip.brynmawr.edu*

"Reglan Side Effects and Withdrawal Symptoms." *TDCenter.* Retrieved November 21, 2010, from *www.tardivedyskinesia.com*

Reid, D. *The Complete Book of Chinese Health and Healing.* (Boston: Shambhala, 1995).

Rister, R. (2008, December 26). "What Is MSG Sensitivity Syndrome?" *Ezine@rticles.* Retrieved September 16, 2010, from *http://ezinearticles.com*

Robert, T. (2010, October 18). "Botox Approved by FDA for Chronic Migraine." *Help for Headaches & Migraine.* Retrieved December 2, 2012, from *www.helpforheadaches.com*

———. (2010, March 28). "Gelstat Migraine, the First OTC Migraine Abortive." *Help for Headaches & Migraine.* Retrieved December 10, 2012, from *www.headaches.about.com*

———. *Living Well with Migraine Disease and Headaches.* (New York: HarperCollins Publishers, 2005).

———. "Review: Migra-Cap." *Help for Headaches & Migraine."* Retrieved June 23, 2011, from *www.helpforheadaches.com*

Roth, J. M., MPT. "Physical Therapy and Migraine Headaches." *Michigan Headache & Neurological Institute.* Retrieved June 9, 2011, from *www.mhni.com*

Rowland, A. Z. "Reiki: Hands on Healing." *Wisdom Magazine's Web Edition.* Retrieved September 8, 2012, from *http://wisdom-magazine.com*

Sahai-Srivastava, S., M.D., and Ko, D.Y., M.D. (2009, December 10). "Pathophysiology and Treatment of Migraine Related Headache." *eMedicine.* Retrieved February 11, 2010, from *http://emedicine.medscape.com*

Sauro, K. M., MSc., and Werner, J. B., M.D., FRCPC. (2009). "The Stress and Migraine Interaction." *Headache: The Journal of Head and Face Pain, 49* (9): 1378–1386.

Schacter, M. B., M.D., FACAM. (2000). "Hypothyroidism." *Schacter Center for Complementary Medicine.* Retrieved February 12, 2010, from *www.mbschacter.com*

Schultz, T. (2010, January 13). "The Five Element Theory in TCM." *emedicnehealth.* Retrieved January 1, 2011, from *www.suite101.com*

Silberstein, S. D., M.D. (2008). "Approach to the Patient with Headache." *Merck Manual of Patient Symptoms.* Retrieved July 27, 2010, from *www.merck.com*

————. (2008, April). "Migraine." *Merck Manual of Patient Symptoms.* Retrieved February 11, 2010, from *www.merck. com*

————. (2008). "Migraines." *Merck Manual Home Edition.* Retrieved September 27, 2010, from *www.merck.com*

Silberstein, S. D., and R. B. Lipton (2004, April). "Migraine and Epilepsy." *Epilepsy.com.* Retrieved February 12, 2010, from *http://professionals.epilepsy.com*

Smith, M. "Discovering Qigong." *Share Guide, The Holistic Health Magazine and Resource Directory.* Retrieved May 31, 2011, from *www.shareguide.com*

Sorgen, C. (2005, January 12). "Exercise Can Be a Pain in the—Head." *WebMD.* Retrieved December 10, 2012, from *www. webmd.com*

Stachowiak, J., PhD. "Headaches as a Symptom of Multiple Sclerosis." *About.com.* Retrieved November 19, 2009, from *http://ms.about.com*

St. John, M. (2003). "Traditional Chinese Medicine—The Five Elements." *acupuncture-online.* Retrieved January 11, 2010, from *www.acupuncture-online.com*

Tao, W. "Chinese Medicine Theory: Pathogenic Factors-1." *damo-qigonng.net*. Retrieved December 10, 2012, from *www. damo-qigong.net*

Tietjen, G. E., et al. (2007). "Endometriosis Is Associated with Prevalence of Comorbid Conditions in Migraine." *Headache, 47* (7): 1069–78.

Treximet. *Everyday Health*. Retrieved December 10, 2012, from *www.everydayhealth.com*

University of Maryland Medical Center. (2008, October 11). "Feverfew." *University of Maryland medical Center*. Retrieved from *www.umm.edu*

———. (2008, September 9). "Migraine Headaches—Medications for Treating Migraine Attacks." *University of Maryland Medical Center*. Retrieved November 27, 2010, from *www.umm.edu*

———. (2008, December 23). "Willowbark." *University of Maryland Medical Center*. Retrieved from *www.umm.edu.*

University of Minnesota. "Healing Touch: Taking Charge of Your Health." Retrieved June 29, 2011, from *www.takingcharge.csh.umn.edu*

———. (2012, June 4). "How Does Reiki Work? Taking Charge of Your Health." Retrieved December 10, 2012, from *www.takingcharge.csh.umn.edu*

University of Montreal. (2010, September 17). "Gene Linked to Common Form of Migraine Discovered." *ScienceDaily*. Retrieved November 5, 2010, from *www.sciencedaily.com*

Vidal, V. O., BS., MA., H(ASCP). "The Role of Stress in Migraine Headache, Serotonin Dysfunction, and the Initiation of Depression." *Outcrybookreview.com*. Retrieved July 14, 2010, from *www.outcrybookreview.com*

Wall Street Journal. (2011, January 05). "Studies Show Botox Can Reduce Migraine Headaches." Retrieved December 10, 2012, from *www.foxnews.com*

Wenzel, R., PharmD. (2010). "Headache Medication Guide." *National Pain Foundation.* Retrieved November 20, 2010, from *www.nationalpainfoundation.org*

Williams, M., ND. (2004). "Health Conditions and Concerns, Headaches—Exercise: A New Migraine Headache Therapy." *Bastyr Center for Natural Health.* Retrieved October 7, 2009, from *http://bastyrcenter.org*

Young, B., M.D., and S. D. Silberstein, M.D. *Migraine and Other Headaches.* (New York: Demos Medical Publishing, 2004).

Zecuity. "Zecuity—Migraine Treatment." Retrieved January 24, 2013, from *www.zecuity.com*

Index

Tables are indicated with *t* following the page number.

A

abdominal migraines, 23
abortive medications, 66, 69, 75–78
acetaminophen, 68, 73
acetylsalicylic acid (aspirin), 69, 73
acupressure, 136–137
acupuncture, 88, 134–136, 143, 170
adrenal glands, 60, 113
Advil, 69
age of onset, 14, 15–16, 19
agitation, 7
alcohol, 36, 44–45, 54, 56, 57, 71
almotriptan, 77
alprazolam, 71
altitude changes, 29, 46, 49
Amerge, 77
American Headache Society Committee for Headache Education (AHS), 168
American Migraine Foundation, 168
amitriptyline, 72, 80
analgesics, 66, 68–72
anger, 108
anorexia, 7
antibiotics, 72, 78
anticonvulsants, 66, 71, 81–82
antidepressants, 72, 78, 80

antiemetics, 66, 74–75
antihistamines, 71
anti-seizure medications, 81
anxiety, 10, 26, 54
appetite changes, 7, 10
artificial sweeteners, 36
aspartame, 36
aspirin, 69, 73
attitude, 114, 173
auras (biofields), 159, 160
auras (pre-headache symptoms), 8–9, 18, 22
autonomic nervous system, 11, 140
Axert, 77

B

Bai shao, 133
Bai zhi, 133
barometric pressure changes, 46
basilar artery migraines, 22–23, 76
beta blockers, 79
beverage triggers
    common, 35–41, 39*t*
    food allergy *vs.*, 35
    identification and management of, 41–46
biofeedback, 155–156
biofields, 159, 160
bipolar disorder, 26, 28
birth control pills, 50, 52
bisoprolol, 79
bladder channel, 91

Blocadren, 79
blood pressure medications, 79–80
blood tests, 19
Botox (botulinum toxin type A),
    81–82
brain tumors, 20, 26
breathing exercises, 47, 140,
    153–155
butorphanol, 70
butterbur, 53, 130

C

Cafergot, 78
caffeine
    in combination medications,
        73, 78
    magnesium levels affected by, 54
    medication absorption assis-
        tance, 74
    as migraine abortive remedy,
        36, 73
    rebound headaches caused by,
        74
    as trigger, 44
    withdrawals from, as trigger,
        56, 57
Calan, 80, 82
calcium channel blockers, 79–80
calendars, 42, 51, 62–64
carbamazepine, 71
cayenne, 132
central nervous system (CNS), 5,
    11–12, 140
Chai hu, 133
chakras, 159, 160, 161
chamomile, 72
channels (meridians), 90–91, 92t,
    134, 136–137, 159
chemicals, 35–38, 43, 52
chi, 89–90, 134, 159

children, 14, 15–16, 23
chiropractic therapy, 150
chlordiazepoxide, 71
chlorpromazine, 74
chocolate, 44. *See also* caffeine
chronic daily headache (CDH), 25
chronic migraines, 22
cigarette smoke, 9, 48
cluster headaches, 17, 25
codeine, 70, 73
coffee. *See* caffeine
cold compresses, as relief method,
    17, 106–017
cold energy, 106–107, 112
cold therapy, 156–157
combination medications, 66, 70,
    73–74, 77
comorbid diseases, 28–30
Compazine, 74
computers, 46, 48
concentration, 7, 10
confusion, 10, 19, 23
constipation, 8
contraceptives, oral, 50, 52
Corgard, 79
cortical spreading depression theory,
    4, 8, 112–113
cortisol, 53, 59, 60
Coumadin, 68, 69, 72, 130
crying, 58
cryotherapy, 156–157
CT scans, 19
cyclobenzaprine, 72

D

dairy, 39, 44
dampness, 105–106, 112
dehydration, 10, 17, 42, 44, 55
Demerol, 70, 72
Depakote, 81

depression, 8, 10, 26, 28

desipramine, 80

DHEA (dehydroepiandrosterone), 60

diagnoses, 14–21, 65–66, 117–124, 119–123*t*

diarrhea, 5, 8, 10

diazepam, 71

diet
    energy networks affected by, 113–114
    food and beverage triggers, common, 35–41, 39–41*t*
    magnesium-rich, 54
    physical triggers and management techniques with, 56–57
    skipped meals, as trigger, 45, 56–57
    Traditional Chinese Medicine and role of, 127–128, 143
    wellness plan development and management of, 42–46, 52, 64, 171–172

dihydroergotamine (DHE), 78

Dilaudid, 70

diphenhydramine, 71

diseases
    comorbid, 28–30
    headaches as symptoms of, 20–21, 25, 26
    medications altered by, 70
    organ network systems imbalances and, 97, 98, 99, 100, 101
    Traditional Chinese Medicine view of, 89, 103–109

divalproex, 81

Dolophine, 70, 72

Dong quai, 133

dopamine, 4, 5, 6, 51, 74–75, 80

dopamine antagonists, 74–75

driving, 48

drowsiness, 8

drugs, 56. *See also* medications

dryness, 106

Du huo, 133

E

earth (element/phase), 94, 95*t*, 96, 119–123*t*

EEGs (electroencephalograms), 15, 19

Effexor, 80

Elavil, 72, 80

elements
    mind-spirit balancing and, 116
    organ network systems and relationship to, 92–94, 95*t*, 96
    TCM examination and migraine diagnoses, 118–124, 119–123*t*

eletriptan (Relpax), 63, 77

elimination diets, 42

emotions, 107–110, 114–116, 161–162, 172

endometriosis, 28, 29

endorphins, 5, 51, 150, 151, 161

energy
    balance of, 90, 137
    chi, 89–90
    emotional, 107–109
    healing therapies using, 159–162
    massage techniques unblocking, 138
    mind-spirit balance, 114–116
    organ network system, 95*t*, 96–102
    phases of, 92–94, 95*t*, 96
    symptoms of blocked channels

heart channel, 91

heart-small intestine network, 97–98, 108

heat, 105, 112

hemicrania continua, 25

hemiplegic migraines, 23, 76

herbs, 53, 67, 72, 129–133, 130–132*t*

HIV medications, 72, 78

homeostasis, 26, 92

hormone replacement therapy (HRT), 50, 52

hormones, 29, 38, 49–53, 59, 60. *See also* epinephrine

hospitalization, 17

hot flashes, 10

hydration, 44–45, 48–49, 57, 172

hydrocodone, 70, 73

hydromorphone, 70

hydroxytryptamine (5-HT), 5. *See also* serotonin

hyperactivity, 7

hypoglycemia, 42

hypothyroidism, 29, 38

I

ibuprofen, 69, 73

imagery, guided, 154–155

imipramine, 80

Imitrex, 18, 63, 69, 77

Inderal, 79

infections, 19, 25

InfiniChi, 137

injections, 67, 77, 81–82

injuries, 21, 25, 26–27, 148–149

integrated theories, 6

integrative therapies
benefits of, 162
biofeedback, 155–156
breathing, 153–155

chiropractic therapy, 150

cold therapy (cryotherapy), 156–157

exercise, 150–151

healing touch, 160–162

introduction and overview, 147–148

massage, 157–158

meditation, 152–153

physical therapy, 148–149

reflexology, 158–159

Reiki, 159–160

resources for, 169–170

wellness plan development for, 163–164, 172

yoga, 152

International Headache Society, 21–26

intestinal channels, 91

irritability, 7, 11

Isoptin, 80

J

Jing jie, 133

joy, 108

Ju hua, 133

K

kava, 72

kidney-bladder network, 101, 113

kidney channel, 92

ko cycles, 96

L

lacrimation (tearing), 10, 23, 25

lemon balm, 72, 132

let down migraines, 61

Librium, 71

lifestyle interference, 17

light, 7, 9, 10, 23, 46, 47, 48

60

testosterone, 53

Tezampanel, 83

thirst, 8

Thorazine, 74

thundercap headaches, 19

thyroid, 29, 38

Tian ma, 133

Tigan, 74

timolol, 79

Tofranil, 80

tongue, diagnostic observations of, 120–121, 121*t*

Topamax, 81

touch sensitivity, 10

Traditional Chinese Medicine (TCM)

  causes of disease, 103–109

  channels and energy flow, 91–92*t*

  chi, 89–90

  introduction, 87–89

  migraine disease and mind-spirit balance, 114–116

  migraine disease and organ network systems, 111–114

  migraine disease diagnosis, 117–124, 119–123*t*

  migraine disease treatments, 127–144

  organ network system, 96–101

  phases/elements of energy, 92–96, 95*t*

  yin and yang balance, 90

travel, 48–49

TRESK, 13, 83

Trexan, 72

Treximet, 77

triggers

  calendar documentation and

  pattern identification, 42, 62–64

  diagnostic questions and associated, 18

  environmental, 46–49

  food and beverage, 34–46, 39–41*t*, 171

  hormonal, 49–53

  introduction, 33–34

  mineral deficiencies as, 53–55

  physical and emotional, 55–58

  stress and susceptibility to, 60–61

trimethobenzamide, 74

triple warmer channel, 92

triptans, 23, 76

Tui Na (Tuina), 138

turmeric, 131

Tylenol (acetaminophen), 68, 73

tyramine, 35, 36

U

unifying theories, 6

urinalysis tests, 19

V

valerian, 132

Valium, 71

valley of harmony, 136–137

vascular system

  altitude and barometric pressure affecting, 46

  cold therapy affecting, 156–157

  diseases of, causing secondary migraines, 25

  environmental triggers affecting, 49

  foods and food ingredients affecting, 35, 36, 37, 39, 44, 73

About the Author

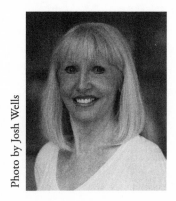

Photo by Josh Wells

Sharron Murray, MS, RN, taught critical care nursing at California State University Long Beach for twenty-five years. She has spoken extensively on topics related to critical care nursing and physical assessments of adults, and has published in numerous professional journals. Visit her at *www.sharronmurray.com*.

Dr. Mao Shing Ni is a 38th generation doctor of Chinese medicine, an authority on Taoist anti-aging medicine, and author of the bestselling book *Secrets of Longevity*.

To Our Readers

Conari Press, an imprint of Red Wheel/Weiser, publishes books on topics ranging from spirituality, personal growth, and relationships to women's issues, parenting, and social issues. Our mission is to publish quality books that will make a difference in people's lives—how we feel about ourselves and how we relate to one another. We value integrity, compassion, and receptivity, both in the books we publish and in the way we do business.

Our readers are our most important resource, and we appreciate your input, suggestions, and ideas about what you would like to see published.

Visit our website at *www.redwheelweiser.com* to learn about our upcoming books and free downloads, and be sure to go to *www.redwheelweiser.com/newsletter* to sign up for newsletters and exclusive offers.

You can also contact us at *info@rwwbooks.com*.

Conari Press
an imprint of Red Wheel/Weiser, LLC
665 Third Street, Suite 400
San Francisco, CA 94107